Positive Health

This comprehensive compendium offers a wealth of research-informed tools that can boost both physical and mental wellbeing throughout the life span. Filled with more than 100 activities to help you live life better, this book is the first of its kind to integrate the latest research from the fields of positive psychology and lifestyle medicine.

Striking a careful balance between theory and practice, the book first reviews what is known about positive psychology and health, presenting a novel approach to holistic wellbeing. It then goes on to provide more than 100 tools designed to increase physical, mental, and social health and wellbeing and also to decrease the risk of illness and disease. The tools described can be used by people of all ages, whether well or experiencing illness. It includes tools that you can use to improve your nutrition and sleep, to increase your physical activity, to develop positive relationships, to develop a positive mindset, and to pursue a meaning in life. These tools provide research-informed, practical advice to help you to make lasting changes and become the best possible version of yourself.

This book is invaluable for anyone who wishes to maintain and enhance their health and wellbeing using tools that have been shown through research to be effective. It is also a key text for students in positive psychology and healthcare, as well as serving as an evidence-based reference book for coaches and health professionals who wish to recommend research-informed tools to their clients and patients.

Jolanta Burke (PhD) is a chartered psychologist specialising in positive psychology and a senior lecturer at the Centre for Positive Psychology and Health, RCSI University of Medicine and Health Sciences. For more information, go to www.jolantaburke.com.

Pádraic J. Dunne (PhD) is an immunologist (research scientist) and accredited psychotherapist with an interest in researched meditation-based interventions for health, managing burnout among healthcare workers, and community-based digital solutions for promoting health and wellbeing.

Trudy Meehan is a chartered clinical psychologist and lecturer at the Centre for Positive Psychology and Health, RCSI University of Medicine and Health Sciences.

Professor Ciaran A. O'Boyle is a psychologist and pharmacologist with a particular interest in the interface between lifestyle medicine and positive psychology. During a long career at the RCSI University of Medicine and Health Sciences, he established the University's Department of Psychology, its Institute of Leadership, and its Centre for Positive Psychology and Health.

Christian van Nieuwerburgh is a professor of coaching and positive psychology at RCSI University of Medicine and Health Sciences, Principal Fellow at the Centre for Wellbeing Science at the University of Melbourne, and global director of Growth Coaching International.

"There is no book on Positive Health that is more readable, applicable, concise, and practical, yet underpinned by rigorous science and the authors' sage wisdom. As a must-read, the book owner will enjoy a delightful guide towards health and happiness."

Associate Professor Aaron Jarden, *Centre for Wellbeing Science, University of Melbourne, Australia*

"This book is a treasure trove of health and wellbeing practices based on current science. I love that this book is for both health care practitioners and professionals and for anyone wanting to improve their health and wellbeing. Given we are so overloaded with competing and often contradictory information on our health and wellbeing, my recommendation is that this book becomes the go-to handbook in your health and wellbeing library."

Dr Suzy Green, *Honorary Professor in the School of Psychology, University of East London, CEO and Founder of the Positivity Institute dedicated to the research and application of Positive Psychology*

"Reading this book is like the awe and magic invoked by apothecaries of old, making incantations, stirring esoteric herbs and body parts of toads. But rest assured, these are rigorous and compassionate scientists who have amassed a Wiki of positive, health inducing actions and experiences. These experiences will stimulate renewal (Parasympathetic Nervous System) which is the only antidote to the ravages of stress. Read it or stay sick!"

Richard Boyatzis, PhD, *Distinguished University Professor, Case Western Reserve University, Co-author of the international best seller* Primal Leadership *and the* New Helping People Change

"The Centre for Positive Psychology and Health at the RCSI University of Medicine and Health Sciences is to be congratulated for their paradigm shifting innovative approach to holistic wellbeing. Their new book now provides the science and evidence (the why), along with actionable support strategies (the how) that enable you to enhance your wellbeing. Whether you are struggling right now, or simply looking at ways to add more life to your years (flourishing in your life, relationships and work), then this book is for you. Read it today, reap lasting benefits and live with more vitality."

Dr Mark Rowe, *Medical Doctor, Waterford, Ireland*

"If you are looking for the gems of well-being – the best habits to be well – look no further. A brilliant team of European experts have mined for you the scientific jewels out of the self-help mountains. They organized the best habits to fit what you are looking for – to feel good, calm down, be energized, find meaning, improve yourself, or connect more with others. Here's to more sparkle and light in our lives."

Margaret Moore, MBA, *Founder/CEO, Wellcoaches Corporation; Co-Founder/Chair, Institute of Coaching, McLean Hospital, Harvard Medical School affiliate; Co-Founder/Board Member, National Board for Health and Wellness Coaching*

"This is a very valuable resource linking the concepts of positive psychology and lifestyle medicine. It provides very user-friendly research-based advice on how to implement positive psychology and health tools into daily life. This book is useful for everyone who needs to bring some positivity into their lives and improve their health. It is especially useful for all involved in education as they may be able to bring some of the learning from the book into their teaching and indirectly impact their students. I loved reading this book and how it introduced me to positive psychology. It is a book that you will go back to time and time again. Every page has some little gem to enhance your day."

Associate Professor Majella Dempsey, *Department of Education, Maynooth University*

"The six pillars of lifestyle medicine include exercise, nutrition, stress resiliency, sleep, social connection, and avoidance of risky substances. Positive psychology comes into play when counselling and coaching patients in all of these pillars. The team at the RCSI University of Medicine and Health Sciences in Dublin has created a pioneering program in Positive Health and their new book is full of science and strategies to help people enjoy enhanced well-being."

Dr. Beth Frates, President-Elect, *American College of Lifestyle Medicine, Faculty Advisor, Harvard Medical School and Director of Lifestyle Medicine and Wellness, Department of Surgery, Massachusetts General Hospital*

Positive Health

100+ Research-Based Positive Psychology and Lifestyle Medicine Tools to Enhance Your Wellbeing

Jolanta Burke
Pádraic J. Dunne
Trudy Meehan
Ciaran A. O'Boyle
Christian van Nieuwerburgh

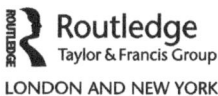

LONDON AND NEW YORK

Cover image: Adobe Stock

First published 2023
by Routledge
4 Park Square, Milton Park, Abingdon, Oxon OX14 4RN

and by Routledge
605 Third Avenue, New York, NY 10158

Routledge is an imprint of the Taylor & Francis Group, an informa business

© 2023 Jolanta Burke, Pádraic J. Dunne, Trudy Meehan, Ciaran A. O'Boyle and Christian van Nieuwerburgh

The right of Jolanta Burke, Pádraic J. Dunne, Trudy Meehan, Ciaran A. O'Boyle and Christian van Nieuwerburgh to be identified as authors of this work has been asserted in accordance with sections 77 and 78 of the Copyright, Designs and Patents Act 1988.

All rights reserved. No part of this book may be reprinted or reproduced or utilised in any form or by any electronic, mechanical, or other means, now known or hereafter invented, including photocopying and recording, or in any information storage or retrieval system, without permission in writing from the publishers.

Trademark notice: Product or corporate names may be trademarks or registered trademarks, and are used only for identification and explanation without intent to infringe.

British Library Cataloguing-in-Publication Data
A catalogue record for this book is available from the British Library

Library of Congress Cataloging-in-Publication Data
A catalog record for this book has been requested

ISBN: 978-1-032-24639-0 (hbk)
ISBN: 978-1-032-24638-3 (pbk)
ISBN: 978-1-003-27959-4 (ebk)

DOI: 10.4324/9781003279594

Typeset in Bembo
by Apex CoVantage

To all our readers. May this book serve you well.

Contents

Centre for Positive Psychology and Health   xii

PART I
Health and wellbeing   1

1 **Introduction**   3
   Before you begin 5
   Positive psychology and health tools 10
   Enhancing health and wellbeing 12
   How to use this book 16

PART II
Health and wellbeing tools   21

2 **Calming tools**   23
   Introduction 23
   Sleep 24
   Meditation 32
   Nature 37
   Creativity 42
   Green care 47
   Your reflection space 50

3 **Energising tools**   51
   Physical activity 52
   Blue spaces 60
   Nutrition 63

Play 68
Humour 73
Your reflection space 78

4 **Coping tools** 79
Expressive writing 80
Optimism 84
Bibliotherapy 89
Stress mindset 93
Compassion 100
Your reflection space 107

5 **Feeling-good tools** 108
Reminiscing 110
Strengths 113
Gratitude 118
Music 122
Art viewing 126
Your reflection space 129

6 **Meaning-making tools** 130
Exploring meaning 131
Positive identity 135
Benefit finding 138
Legacy (scarcity) 143
Photography 146
Your reflection space 149

7 **Relationship tools** 150
Capitalisation 151
Forgiveness 153
Kindness 156
Savouring relationships 161
Your reflection space 166

8 **Prospecting** 167
Anticipation 168
Goal setting 173
Best possible self 175
Hope 179
Your reflection space 183

                                                    Contents   xi

9 **Emerging tools and concepts**   184
   Storytelling 184
   Self-care 185
   Social media 187
   Self-reassurance 189

PART III
Making a lasting change   195

10 **Going with the waves of change**   197
   Reflection time 202
   Making positive change happen 202
   Health plan 203
   Use a coaching framework 204
   Find a coach 209
   Find a therapist 209
   Conclusion 212

   Index   213

Centre for Positive Psychology and Health

The Centre for Positive Psychology and Health at the RCSI University of Medicine and Health Sciences was established in 2019 in response to the increasing prevalence of diseases associated with lifestyle and the growing evidence for the role of psychological factors in optimising health and wellbeing. Our mission is to educate, nurture, and discover to enhance health and wellbeing through positive psychology, positive organisational scholarship, and lifestyle medicine.

We consider public engagement to be central to our mission, and we have therefore created a series of free massive open online courses (MOOC): The Science of Health and Happiness, The Science of Health and Happiness for Young People, and The Science of Health and Happiness as We Age. Our courses have already attracted over 30,000 participants in the first year. Please visit the RCSI University webpage (see below) for further details.

Given the importance of scientific evidence for healthcare interventions, please visit our public engagement and support webpage for additional, up-to-date, validated resources aimed to help you enhance your wellbeing.

Centre for Positive Psychology and Health webpage: www.rcsi.com/dublin/about/faculty-of-medicine-and-health-sciences/centre-for-positive-psychology-and-health.

Part I
Health and wellbeing

1 Introduction

We all aspire to being healthy and happy. However, the prevalence of diseases such as cancer, heart disease, stroke, diabetes, and mental illness continues to rise in both the developed and developing worlds. These noncommunicable diseases (NCDs) kill 41 million people each year, equivalent to 71% of all deaths globally (WHO, 2021a). Almost a million people a year commit suicide, and this has become the fourth leading cause of death for teenagers (WHO, 2021b). Many of us who are not suffering from such diseases would accept that while we are not ill, we are not flourishing either. The COVID pandemic has certainly played a role here, and many of us find ourselves stuck in a limbo that some researchers in the past have called *"languishing"* (Keyes, 2002).

Our health and wellbeing are determined by a whole range of complex interactions between such factors as our genetic makeup, our environment, our socioeconomic grouping, our early childhood experiences, our employment status, our health literacy, and our own behaviours (Egger et al., 2017). While many of these factors are beyond our control, the good news is that research has shown that by controlling what have become known as lifestyle factors, we can prevent disease, enhance our health and wellbeing, and extend our lives (Egger et al., 2017; Frates et al., 2019; Kelly & Clayton, 2021; Kenny, 2022; Swann et al., 2010). Clearly, we won't always be able to offset the effects of such external factors as poverty, social exclusion, and lack of access to adequate health services, but many of us will be able to improve our health and wellbeing through our own efforts.

According to the WHO, one of the most important ways of reducing deaths and disease burden from NCDs is to control unhealthy lifestyle choices that lead to their development. Strategies include reducing the use of tobacco and the harmful use of alcohol, maintaining an active lifestyle, and developing a healthy diet. It is estimated that up to 80% of cases of coronary heart disease, 90% of type 2 diabetes cases, and one-third of cancers could be avoided by changing to a healthier diet, increasing physical activity, and stopping smoking (WHO, 2021d). We also know from a large body of research that there is much we can do proactively to improve our mental health and to increase our levels of happiness (Carr, 2020).

In this book, we have curated a compendium of research-based tools to help you make discerning choices about improving your health and wellbeing. All the tools presented here have been developed by researchers who specialise in this area, and all of them have been subjected to experimental studies to ensure their effectiveness. While this does not mean that every tool will work for every individual – one's preferences are just as unique as one's DNA – it should be possible for you to find at least some tools that will work for you.

This is the first practitioner-focused book that amalgamates wellbeing and health research. It is intended to be used by healthcare practitioners seeking additional ways to support their clients and also by members of the general public setting out to improve their health and wellbeing. It is a topic that we, the authors, are passionate about. We share a deep commitment to the enhancement of wellbeing, both personally and professionally. This text should be useful for healthcare professionals, coaches, consultants, and individuals who want to consider a range of research-informed practices and interventions designed to enhance health and wellbeing. But most importantly, it should be beneficial for any human being, younger or older, going through a challenging period or enjoying their lives, in sickness or in health – a person interested in using research-informed practices to enhance their health and wellbeing.

When used with clients, we advocate a "coaching approach" to selecting interventions and designing wellbeing plans. This means that health professionals, coaches, doctors, etc. would prefer listening to their clients, working with them to identify suitable interventions and co-constructing wellbeing plans, rather than simply prescribing a way forward.

The "wellness" industry has grown exponentially in recent years and is now estimated to be worth $1.5 trillion per annum (Remes et al., 2020). This has led to a bewildering array of methods, tools, and advice, much of it unsupported by scientific research. In this book, we have drawn heavily on the new science of positive psychology and on the rapidly developing specialty of lifestyle medicine. We have also made sure that the tools selected have been tested in clinical and non-clinical populations, thus helping a person to select a range of wellbeing tools that can be used in various stages of one's life, whether one is healthy or unwell. We hope that this book can support individuals on their recovery or wellness journey, regardless of their circumstances.

Before you begin

Let us discuss a few essential points to help you understand how using this book can assist you in enhancing your health and wellbeing. We will first clarify what we mean by health and wellbeing, then delve into some research relating to health and wellbeing and set out what you need to know about using the tools we have compiled. Finally, we will provide guidance on how best to use this book.

What do we mean by "health" and "wellbeing"?

We often talk about "health" and "wellbeing" in one breath. However, both are complex constructs and mean different things to different people. An extensive literature review of texts on health and wellbeing identified a nuanced relationship between them (Pelters, 2021). "Health" is sometimes viewed as an umbrella term that includes wellbeing. Alternatively, the two terms are sometimes used synonymously, or they are viewed as independent. Some researchers consider health to be a more objective concept, with wellbeing seen as a more subjective concept that depends on individuals' psychological processes.

The World Health Organisation (WHO) usefully defines health as "a state of complete physical, mental and social well-being and not merely the absence of disease or infirmity". Health is seen as "a resource for everyday life, not the objective of living". Here, health is seen as a positive concept emphasizing social and personal resources as well as physical capacities. The WHO defines mental health as "a state of well-being in which every individual realizes his or her own potential, can cope with the normal stresses of life, can work productively and fruitfully, and is able to make a contribution to her or his community" (WHO, 2021c).

Important conclusions can be drawn from these definitions.

1 Health is more than the absence of disease. Most "health services" are designed to treat illness and disease rather than to enhance health in the wider sense of the term as used here. Many of us see health and disease as binary – we are healthy when we are not ill and vice versa (Figure 1.1). However, the WHO definition underpins the fact that there is more to being healthy than simply not being ill. Heretofore, medical and psychological interventions were largely designed to restore health, in the sense of treating illness. Thus, for example, the treatment objective in patients with depression is usually to help them move from experiencing depression to *not* experiencing any symptoms of depression. However, interventions are less likely to be

6 *Health and wellbeing*

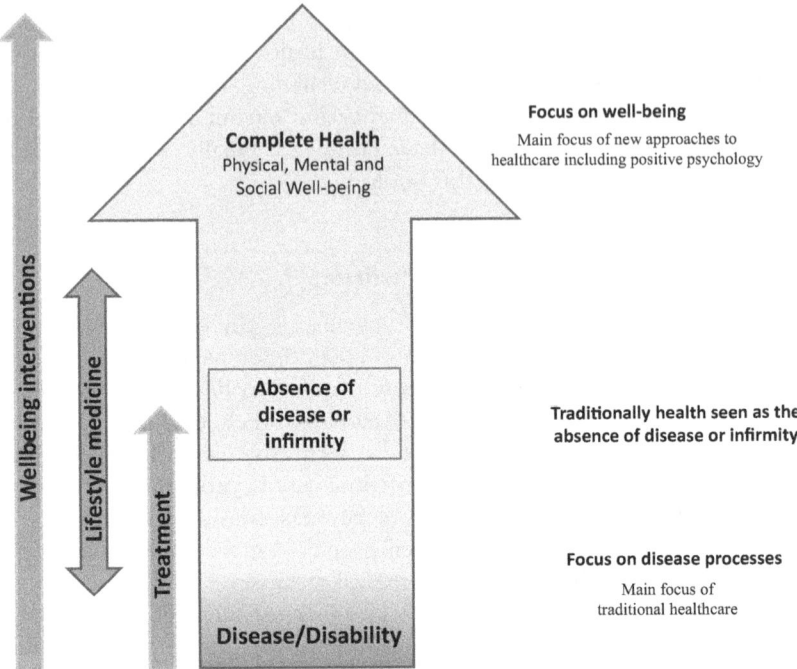

Figure 1.1 Approaches to health and well-being. Traditionally health has been seen as the absence of disease, and most treatments as designed to return patient to this state. More wholistic approaches to health (including the WHO approach) are concerned with treatment and prevention, but also focus on upper section of the model i.e. helping everyone to achieve complete health which is seen as a state of complete well-being and not merely the absence of disease or infirmity. Lifestyle medicine is mainly concerned with reducing risk and with prevention but interventions also move people towards complete health which includes physical, mental and social well-being. Positive psychology also contributes here by focusing on the enabling everyone to live happy and meaningful lives.

designed to extend or develop broader health assets such as strengths, optimism, and growth mindsets. By the end of the series of treatments, clients may not be sick but not fully healthy either in terms of the broad definition of complete health advanced by the WHO.

2   The WHO definition identifies three crucial components of health: physical, mental, and social. It can be argued that our approaches to healthcare have, in the past, focused more on physical health than mental health and more on both of these than on social health. It follows from the WHO definition that it is possible to have a physical disease and yet experience good levels of mental and/or social health.

Conversely, one can be physically well but suffer poor mental and/or social health (Keyes, 2002). A large research literature exists demonstrating the relative independence of physical disease and subjective quality of life. Research with over 6,000 people in the UK showed that 35% of them experienced both symptoms of illness (e.g. depression) and wellbeing (e.g. high levels of self-esteem), thus suggesting that, even in mental illness, some features of wellbeing can co-exist (Huppert & Whittington, 2003).

3   Rather than focusing exclusively on disease and illness, healthcare could focus on maximising the health (in its fullest sense) of everyone, the goal being to support everyone to flourish. This broad notion of flourishing is not one that many people immediately think about when they think about health. Many of the tools discussed in this book have been designed to help you improve your health in the broader sense of the term being used here.

Can our attitudes and behaviour change our genes?

Many people believe that their health, wellbeing, and longevity are determined largely by their genes. There is no doubt that our genetic makeup has important consequences for us, but the key question is the extent of that influence and how it might be altered. Modern research has established that our genes can be switched on and off by factors such as diet, exercise, and our psychological approach and attitude to life. This emerging field of study is called epigenetics, and it implies that we can influence the expression of our genes in both positive and negative ways. This interaction between our environment and our genes is complex and differs between individuals.

The key lifestyle influencers on our genes are diet, physical activity, smoking and alcohol consumption, sleep habits, chronic stress, and conditions such as obesity, infections, and exposure to environmental chemical contaminants (Panico et al., 2021). The manner in which we age is also influenced by our genes, but here again, lifestyle factors and psychological processes can alter the rate of ageing. Perceptions of ageing, feelings of control, and emotional responses to getting older are important factors. A positive attitude towards ageing changes cell chemicals in a beneficial manner, possibly by reducing inflammation in the cells and thereby changing gene expression (Kenny, 2022).

Some people claim that they have a "grumpy gene" or complain they have inherited depression and other mental health disorders from their parents. Such views were influenced by a limited number of research studies published in the 1980s and 1990s. Recent studies have established that approximately 78% of our wellbeing can be attributed to factors in our environment (Bartels, 2015). Individuals differ in terms of their sensitivity to the environment (Pluess et al., 2018). In a study evaluating the effectiveness of a resilience programme, researchers found that some individuals' wellbeing changed significantly immediately after the programme and the effects continued at follow-up. In contrast, other participants experienced a much smaller change in their wellbeing and were more likely to return to baseline at follow-up (Pluess & Boniwell, 2015). People with high sensitivity can "travel" on the wellbeing spectrum more easily than others. Thus, for some of you, this book could be a source of significant enhancement in health and wellbeing, whereas others might not be impacted to the same extent.

The key message is that your genes are not your destiny. Your lifestyle is your destiny. The changes you make today will change your lifestyle and ultimately change your future (Kelly & Clayton, 2021).

Positive psychology, lifestyle medicine, and health

In this book, we take a unique perspective on health, drawing mainly from the science of positive psychology (Carr, 2020; Schui & Krampen, 2010) and the rapidly developing specialty of lifestyle medicine (Egger et al., 2017; Frates et al., 2019). In addition, we have also drawn, but to a lesser extent, from some of the findings in health psychology (Ogden, 2019), clinical psychology (Carr, 2016), and integrative medicine (Rakel, 2018). All these approaches to healthcare are based on the idea that solutions to preventing disease and promoting health should be a collaborative process between provider and patient or client. A substantial value is placed on the therapeutic alliance between the two parties. Many of the tools described in this book, such as eating well, taking exercise, and maximising sleep hygiene, are increasingly being prescribed by healthcare practitioners. Of course, many of the tools derived from these approaches can be used by individuals themselves without recourse to formal medical or psychological healthcare systems.

By enhancing our health and wellbeing, we are also affecting the wellbeing of our loved ones, the people we interact with daily, our neighbours, friends, colleagues, and potentially even strangers. Therefore, investing in one's health and wellbeing is not a selfish act. Minding ourselves creates a ripple effect that affects our entire community. If we are not doing it for ourselves, let us do it for others!

Positive psychology is a relatively new approach in psychology that focuses on the conditions for human flourishing (Seligman & Csikszentmihalyi, 2000). Traditionally, psychological research had focused almost exclusively on the negative aspects of human experience such as stress, illness, and all that prevents us from being the best versions of ourselves. For example, by 1998, 17 out of 18 published studies in psychology focused on depression as opposed to wellbeing (Achor, 2010). In neuroscience, nine out of ten (93%) of studies focused on cognitive decline instead of cognitive health (Randolph, 2013). By 2011, barely 3% of research in public health focused on the positive aspects of health (Rusk & Waters, 2013). This means that over a century, we have gained more knowledge about being *un*happy, experiencing dementia, and other diseases than about being well and thriving, physically, mentally, and socially.

Early advocates of positive psychology called for an increase in research about the positive aspects of human beings and their lives. They were interested in ways in which we could use our strengths and other resources to help us function at an optimal level. Research under the umbrella of positive psychology considers our positive attributes, states, behaviours, attitudes, etc. as unique entities worthy of empirical exploration in their own right. It also encourages research that examines health factors, especially those relating to the optimal aspects of health, such as psychological flourishing. Finally, it provides an array of interventions that aim to support individuals in experiencing optimum health.

Our starting point when we came to write this book was to try to help the majority of people who are well develop their positive assets and experience a higher level of wellbeing or at least maintain their current levels of wellbeing. However, given that positive psychology interventions have also been used to help people who experience mental health issues, such as depression or anxiety (e.g. Bolier et al., 2013), the tools described here can also be useful for those who are unwell.

One of the most significant criticisms of positive psychology has been that it largely disregarded physiological and physical aspects of human flourishing. As one critic put it, positive psychology saw human beings as floating heads (Hefferon, 2013). This is where research in the developing field of lifestyle medicine can complement positive psychology. Lifestyle medicine is the application of medical, behavioural, motivational, and environmental principles to the management of lifestyle-related health problems in clinical settings (Egger et al., 2017). Teaching self-care and self-management are important elements of lifestyle medicine. Lifestyle medicine focuses on six areas that improve health and prevent disease (Frates et al., 2021):

1 Healthful eating of whole, plant-based foods
2 Physical activity
3 Stress management
4 Forming and maintaining relationships

5   Sleep improvement
6   Avoiding risky substances

In this book, we have sought to complement the tools derived from positive psychology, which focus largely on psychological wellbeing, with a range of interventions drawn from lifestyle medicine, which tend to focus more on health behaviours.

Positive psychology and health tools

What differentiates positive psychology from other disciplines is the robust range of tools the researchers have developed aimed specifically at enhancing wellbeing. These are referred to as positive psychology interventions (PPIs) and are defined as techniques one can use to bolster positive feelings, behaviours, and thinking (Sin & Lyubomirsky, 2009). These interventions can consist of brief self-administered practices or longer-term programmes comprising a range of tools. While many of these methods focus on changing individuals' emotions (e.g. savouring the moment) and thinking (e.g. *thinking* grateful thoughts), a limited number of them also focus on amending behaviours (e.g. asking participants to *perform* acts of kindness) that result in positive outcomes. A more comprehensive definition of PPIs states that "the goal of each tool is to build positive elements, providing evidence that deems the tool research-based and that evidence demonstrates positive outcomes" (Parks & Biswas-Diener, 2013). In selecting tools for this book, we have followed these criteria, ensuring that all the tools we included have evidence of positive outcomes.

We have also included a range of tools developed in the context of lifestyle medicine. Many of these focus on reducing risk by changing health-related behaviours, and many incorporate findings from the discipline of health psychology. Such interventions provide people with more control over their health and have been shown to be effective approaches in prevention and treatment (Kelly & Clayton, 2021).

Tool inclusion criteria

When searching the literature for the most appropriate tools to include here, we applied three inclusion criteria. Each tool we included provided evidence for all three outcomes:

1   Positive outcome, i.e. enhancing various aspects of health and wellbeing that contribute to psychological flourishing, e.g. self-esteem, engagement, positive emotions, and . . .

2   Reducing illness (mental and physical)
3   Both psychological and physiological effects on wellness (Figure 1.2)

Given the wide range of interventions claimed to enhance wellbeing, it is important to establish an evidence base for an intervention rather than relying on anecdote. In selecting tools for this book, we sought scientific evidence that they had been assessed and validated in at least one experimental research study. Some of the tools have a more extensive evidence base than others, but all of them have been subjected to at least some experimental validation.

The nature of research is such that many of the tools described have been studied using a particular methodology and in a particular cohort of subjects. It follows that strict scientific evidence for the generalisability of many of them is still somewhat limited. In addition, positive psychology and lifestyle medicine are still young disciplines, and with time, more evidence and greater refinement of these tools will emerge.

In positive psychology, many tools have been assessed as part of multi-tool programmes (Rashid & Seligman, 2019), and it can be difficult to ascertain the specific effectiveness of any one tool in isolation. This means, for example, that we know that a programme that includes a "positive legacy activity" enhances wellbeing, but we do not know if this specific activity has the same effect on its own. Some activities that were originally included in multi-tool programmes have since been tested individually. For example, the technique "One door closes, another door opens", part of the Penn Resiliency programme, was subsequently tested by Gander et al. (2013). In this book, we included only a handful of tools tested as part of wellbeing programmes on each occasion, highlighting that they were not assessed on their own.

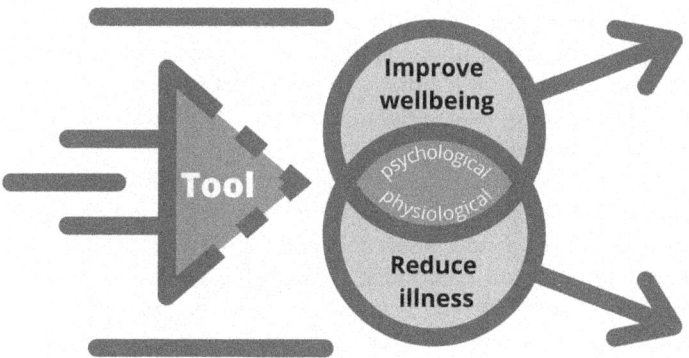

Figure 1.2 Types of positive psychology and health tools.

Whereas we have sought to adopt strict scientific criteria in selecting the tools included in this book, we have taken a pragmatic approach in our recommendations about how the tools might be used. For example, using strict scientific criteria, a tool can only be recommended if it is used in precisely the same way it was applied in the studies that provided an evidence base for it. However, in terms of practical application, this is too limiting, and we recommend that you experiment with the tools provided and find what works best for you.

In a similar vein, we did not want to ignore some of the promising correlational research evidence for new psychological and physiological concepts that may be important for increasing health and wellbeing. While not yet meeting the strict empirical criteria we set for the selection of tools, we have, however, included some discussion of these emerging approaches in Chapter 9.

Enhancing health and wellbeing

Enhancing health and wellbeing can be a challenging task. The good news is that we can learn from past research and avoid making unnecessary mistakes. Here is a list of research-informed advice to help you enhance your health and wellbeing.

1. Catch and keep

Wellbeing is not something we catch and keep. Instead, it is something that alters throughout our lives. We may experience a boost of happiness due, for example, to getting married or winning the lottery, but soon, we adapt to our happier life and need more to sustain our happiness (Bao & Lyubomirsky, 2013). We may feel content with our lives until something traumatic suddenly happens which shatters our beliefs. Our wellbeing fluctuates, and just like with exercise, we need to keep at it if we want to be fit. Hedonic adaptation (getting used to whatever made us happy and returning to levels of happiness experienced before the happy event) means that enhancing wellbeing and happiness are not destinations but, rather, a process we go through.

There are two ways to use this book to enhance your wellbeing. Firstly, you can use it in a preventative way, whereby you regularly review the activities, create a plan, and ensure it becomes part of your life. For example, once a month, you could flick through the book and decide which activities you would like to try over the next 4 weeks. This will ensure that you monitor your health and wellbeing, and it may also help you build psychological resources for the future. Secondly, you may choose to use the book as an intervention when something negative happens in your life or when you realise you have not been feeling well recently; you may dust the book off and pick out a series of activities that will help pick you up. Whatever you do, make sure it suits you and that it is having a positive impact.

2. Select tools you enjoy

Whenever you select your tools, make sure you enjoy them. If you have fun using them or find them particularly meaningful, you will be more likely to continue using them. In one experiment, researchers tested a range of activities and found that often, a specific tool seemed to have had a lasting effect on a participant's wellbeing (Seligman et al., 2005). It was easy to assume that it was the best activity for improving wellbeing. However, on further examination, it was found that when participants enjoyed an activity, they persisted in its use after the experiment ended; hence their long-term results. If you find tools you enjoy, you are more likely to continue to use them in the longer term.

3. Select tools that are meaningful to you

Recent research has shown that people found it hard to continue using tools that did not align with their values (Michel et al., 2020). Ensure that the tools you use feel "right" to you. You may find some tools to be too complicated for you. Do not dismiss them too quickly, but try to challenge your views, perhaps tweak them slightly, and try them anyway. Challenging yourself can be helpful in the long term.

4. Tweak the research-based tools

There are over 100 research-based tools and an additional 100+ variations of practice described in this book. Many tools have been tested on research populations that might not reflect your circumstances. Most research has been conducted with college students, although we specifically searched for tools that have been tested with a broader range of participants. The most practical advice we can give is, first, to try out the tools as they are described, and if they work for you, continue to use them in this way; if not, tweak them and make them your own.

5. Don't give up your current wellbeing practice

You may have developed your own health and wellbeing practices and find that they work for you. Having read this book, you may realise, however, that they are not evidence based. This does not mean you should stop your practice. Many daily practices that maintain our wellbeing and health can be challenging to research empirically. "Play" is an example of this; there is a lot of theoretical and neuropsychological support for the idea that play is critical and beneficial not just for children but also for adults. However, this is an area that does not receive large amounts of research funding and, consequently, has a limited amount of research evidence to support the practice.

Another issue to consider is that despite not having a strong evidence base, your preferred practices might be meaningful to you. This "meaning effect" (Moerman & Jonas, 2002) can positively impact healing. We see this, for example with placebos, where belief in the impact of an inert substance can cause physiological and psychological changes. Whilst it is important to be aware of any potential harm that could come from daily practice, it is also wise to consider the personal value a practice adds to your life and the meaning it has for you before you decide to exclude it from your activities.

6. Adopt an open-minded attitude

Whilst we have been careful to select research-informed or evidence-based interventions, the academic field of positive psychology is still young, and further research is needed to understand precisely how and why some of these interventions work. As with other scientific disciplines, we want to be clear at the outset that these interventions are effective in some people in some contexts, so they will not have the expected effect for everyone in every situation. For this reason, we advise an experimental and open-minded attitude to the interventions we have proposed.

7. Vary your activities

It is crucial to vary your activities because you will constantly adapt to them, and as soon as you do, they will stop having the same positive impact on you. You may also sometimes just become bored with them (Sheldon et al., 2013). If you find yourself losing interest and motivation, put the activity back on a shelf and select another one (you have plenty to choose from). Then, a few weeks later, you may pick it up again and re-engage with it. In the meantime, enjoy doing something different.

8. Get social

We are 30 times more likely to smile when in a social situation than when alone (Provine, 2004). Being with people, feeling supported, or supporting others are components of all the main wellbeing models (Burke, 2020). You can amplify the positive impact of all the tools in this book by making them more social. Try inviting friends and colleagues to participate in them with you (Bao & Lyubomirsky, 2014).

9. Get the dosage right

Dosage refers to the frequency with which you use the tools and the number of tools you use at a time. Research establishing the efficacy of a particular tool will have been based on a specific combination and timing regimen. It is best to start with this, but, being pragmatic, you may want to vary the combinations and timing to find a regimen that works best for you. For example if, after selecting five tools or more a week, you stop doing them altogether, then the next week you might select one to three tools and see how you get on with them. Try changing your regimen based on your results. For some activities, such as acts of kindness, the schedule is important. Research has shown that doing several acts of kindness in one day is more effective in boosting wellbeing than spreading them across the week. Therefore, make your own choices about your regimen based on your experiences, the outcomes, and the guidance given for each tool.

10. Keep going

We experience life at different rates; we mature at different paces, depending on our experiences and our biology. What works now might not work in the future and vice versa. We have seen this in a psychotherapeutic context where a young person, for example, is not yet ready to engage in practices like meditation. However, just a few years later, the same person can get great value from meditative-like practices. Remember that agitated brains, minds, and bodies do not always do well initially with calming tools, counselling, and coaching. This is very much the case for those suffering from trauma.

Sometimes, you will have to work on your body first to get it into a position where you will accept calming tools or where these tools will have a positive impact. For example, you might have to alter your diet and adopt an exercise programme before trying yoga or meditation. However, the bottom line is that you come to each tool described in this book with a foundation of compassion for yourself as a human being.

If, after reading this book, you set up your health plan, and a week or two into it, you stop doing it, don't worry, start the next day or the following week again. We all fail. We all make mistakes. We are complex beings. It is possible to be an excellent student one moment and neglect your studies the next day. This is what it means to be a person. This book is for life. You can pick it up and put it down any time you want. If it does not work for you today, maybe you are not ready for it yet. Be gentle with yourself while attempting to maintain your discipline. Remember what Samuel Beckett said: "Ever tried. Ever failed. No matter. Try again. Fail again. Fail better".

11. Adopt a positive attitude

When you believe that these activities will help you enhance your health and wellbeing, you are more likely to see a change. When researchers replicated one of the classic studies in positive psychology (Seligman et al., 2005) with a more sceptical group of people, the results were not as robust (Mongrain & Anselmo-Matthews, 2012). The more open you are to the possibility of wellbeing improvement, the more these tools can help you. If all else fails, remember that they have been effective with others. If they were able to enhance their wellbeing, chances are you will be able to as well.

How to use this book

This book consists of three parts. In Part I, we define health and wellbeing and set out the context for applying personal strategies and taking control of your health and wellbeing. In Part II, we detail over 100 research-based tools you can choose from to enhance your health and wellbeing. In Part III, we discuss research-based tips for successfully embedding these tools in your life and for facilitating meaningful change. This is why we suggest that you read Parts I and III carefully and re-read them when necessary.

Part II, which is the largest part, can be read as a reference book. You can skim-read the eight chapters ("Calming tools", "Energising tools", "Coping tools", "Feeling-good tools", "Meaning-making tools", "Relationship tools", "Prospecting", "Emerging tools and concepts"). Each chapter offers you a brief introduction to its content.

Within each chapter, you will find six sections. Each describes a tool or a group of tools that have been shown to enhance health and wellbeing. The six sections are as follows:

1 **Introduction:** this will help you understand the concepts underpinning the tools described in the
2 **Research-based tools:** these are the tools that have been developed from experimental research.

3   **Variations of practice:** this provides you with additional promising tools — these are tools that are either emerging or tools we have used with our clients and found to be effective, although they need more rigorous scientific examination to fully establish their use. These additional tools bring the total tools offered to you in this book to over 200.
4   **Check out other tools in this book:** this section lists other tools in this book that are in some way connected with a tool you are reading about and, as such, can be used to expand your practice.
5   **Mental and physical health benefits:** here, we provide a brief outline of the evidence we have for the effectiveness of a particular tool. We describe the outcomes of the studies from which the tools emerged and provide additional details of experimental and other studies that help you understand which tools are most suitable for you.
6   **Caveat:** this is an integral part of each tool description that describes where you need to be cautious in using a particular tool. Please make sure you read it before engaging with the tools. Also, note that this section is not exhaustive, and there may be other reasons to be cautious in using or over-using a tool.

Browse through all the activities and decide which ones you feel like practising. First, you can skim-read them; then, when you select a specific chapter or section, you can go deeper into it and re-read it carefully. Make this book your own, highlight your favourite sections, earmark the activities you want to access regularly.

In Part III, we provide you with suggestions of other ways to use this book. You can use it as a one-off resource or a regular guide to enhancing your wellbeing. Alternatively, you can keep the book on your bedside table and read, practise, or plan to do one activity per evening. The most important thing is that you make this book your own. After all, it aims to enhance *your* health and wellbeing, and you know yourself best. Enjoy the journey!

References

Achor, S. (2010). *The happiness advantage: The seven principles that fuel success and performance at work*. Virgin Books.

Bao, K. J., & Lyubomirsky, S. (2013). Making it last: Combating hedonic adaptation in romantic relationships. *The Journal of Positive Psychology, 8*(3), 196–206. https://doi-org.elib.tcd.ie/10.1080/17439760.2013.777765

Bao, K. J., & Lyubomirsky, S. (2014). Making happiness last: Using the hedonic adaptation prevention model to extend the success of positive interventions. In A. C. Parks & S. M. Schueller (Eds.), *The Wiley Blackwell handbook of positive psychological interventions* (pp. 373–384). Wiley Blackwell. https://doi-org.elib.tcd.ie/10.1002/9781118315927.ch21

Bartels, M. (2015). Genetics of wellbeing and its components satisfaction with life, happiness, and quality of life: A review and meta-analysis of heritability studies. *Behavioural Genetics, 45*, 137–156. https://doi.org/10.1007/s10519-015-9713-y

Bolier, L., Haverman, M., Westerhof, G. J., Riper, H., Smit, F., & Bohlmeijer, E. (2013). Positive psychology interventions: A meta-analysis of randomized controlled studies. *BMC Public Health, 13*, 119. https://doi-org.elib.tcd.ie/10.1186/1471-2458-13-119

Burke, J. (2020). *The ultimate guide to implementing wellbeing programmes for school*. Routledge.

Carr, A. (2016). *The handbook of adult clinical psychology: An evidence-based practice approach*. Routledge.

Carr, A. (2020). *Positive psychology and you. A self-development guide*. Routledge.

Egger, G., Binns, A., Rosser, S., & Sagner, M. (2017). *Lifestyle medicine* (3rd ed.). Academic Press.

Frates, B., Bonnet, J. P., Joseph, J., & Peterson, J. A. (2019). *Lifestyle medicine handbook: An introduction to the power of healthy habits*. Healthy Learning.

Frates, B., Bonnet, J. P., Joseph, R., & Peterson, M. A. (2021). *Lifestyle medicine handbook: An introduction to the power of healthy habits* (2nd ed.). Healthy Learning.

Gander, F., Proyer, R. T., Ruch, W., & Wyss, T. (2013). Strength-based positive interventions: Further evidence for their potential in enhancing well-being and alleviating depression. *Journal of Happiness Studies, 14*, 1241–1259. https://doi.org/10.1007/s10902-012-9380-0

Hefferon, K. (2013). *Positive psychology and the body: The somatopsychic side to flourishing*. McGraw Hill Education.

Huppert, F. A., & Whittington, J. E. (2003). Evidence for the independence of positive and negative well-being: Implications for quality of life assessment. *British Journal of Health Psychology, 8*(Pt 1), 107–122. https://doi.org/10.1348/135910703762879246

Kelly, J., & Clayton, J. S. (2021). *Foundations of lifestyle medicine: Board review manual* (3rd ed.). U.S. American College of Lifestyle Medicine.

Kenny, R. A. (2022). *Age proof: The new science of living a longer and healthier life*. Lagon.

Keyes, C. M. (2002). The mental health continuum: From languishing to flourishing in life. *Journal of Health and Social Behavior, 43*(2), 207–222.

Michel, T., Tachtler, F., Slovak, P., & Fitzpatrick, G. (2020). Young people's attitude toward positive psychology interventions: Thematic analysis. *JMIR Human Factors, 7*(4). https://doi-org.elib.tcd.ie/10.2196/21145

Moerman, D. E., & Jonas, W. B. (2002). Deconstructing the placebo effect and finding the meaning response. *Annals of Internal Medicine, 136*(6), 471–476.

Mongrain, M., & Anselmo-Matthews, T. (2012). Do positive psychology exercises work? A Replication of Seligman et al. *Journal of Clinical Psychology, 68*(4), 382. N.PAG. https://doi-org.elib.tcd.ie/10.1002/jclp.21839

Ogden, J. (2019). *Health psychology* (6th ed.). McGrow Hill.

Panico, A., Tumulo, M. R., Leo, C. G. et al. (2021). The influence of lifestyle factors on miRNA expression and signal pathways: A review. *Epigenomics*, *13*(2), 145–164.

Parks, A. C., & Biswas-Diener, R. (2013). Positive interventions: Past, present, and future. In T. B. Kashdan & J. Ciarrochi (Eds.), *Mindfulness, acceptance, and positive psychology: The seven foundations of well-being* (pp. 140–165). Context Press/New Harbinger Publications.

Pelters, P. (2021). Right by your side? – the relational scope of health and wellbeing as congruence, complement and coincidence. *International Journal of Qualitative Studies on Health & Well-Being*, *16*(1), 1–21. https://doi-org.elib.tcd.ie/10.1080/17482631.2021.1927482

Pluess, M., Assary, E., Lionetti, F., Lester, K. J., Krapohl, E., Aron, E. N., & Aron, A. 2018. Environmental sensitivity in children: Development of the highly sensitive child scale and identification of sensitivity groups. *Developmental Psychology*, *54*, 51–70.

Pluess, M., & Boniwell, I. 2015. Sensory-processing sensitivity predicts treatment response to a school-based depression prevention program: Evidence of vantage sensitivity. *Personality and Individual Differences*, *82*, 40–45.

Provine, R. R. (2004). Laughing, tickling, and the evolution of speech and self. *Current Directions in Psychological Science*, *13*(6), 215–218. https://doi.org/10.1111/j.0963-7214.2004.00311.x

Rakel, D. (2018). *Integrative medicine* (4th ed.). Elsevier.

Randolph, J. J. (2013). *Positive neuropsychology: Evidence-based perspectives on promoting cognitive health*. Springer.

Rashid, T., & Seligman, M. E. P. (2019). *Positive psychotherapy: Workbook*. Oxford University Press.

Remes, J., Linzer, K., Singhal, S., et al. (2020). *Prioritising health: A prescription for prosperity*. McKinsey Global Reports. www.mckinsey.com/industries/healthcare-systems-and-services/our-insights/prioritizing-health-a-prescription-for-prosperity

Rusk, R. D., & Waters, L. E. (2013). Tracing the size, reach, impact, and breadth of positive psychology. *The Journal of Positive Psychology*, *8*(3), 207–221. https://doi-org.elib.tcd.ie/10.1080/17439760.2013.777766

Schui, G., & Krampen, G. (2010). Bibliometric analyses on the emergence and present growth of positive psychology. *Applied Psychology: Health & Well-Being*, *2*(1), 52–64. https://doi-org.elib.tcd.ie/10.1111/j.1758-0854.2009.01022.x

Seligman, M. E. P., & Csikszentmihalyi, M. (2000). Positive psychology: An introduction. *American Psychologist*, *55*(1), 5–14. https://doi-org.elib.tcd.ie/10.1037/0003-066X.55.1.5

Seligman, M. E. P., Steen, T. A., Park, N., & Peterson, C. (2005). Positive psychology progress: Empirical validation of interventions. *American Psychologist*, *60*(5), 410–421. https://doi.org/10.1037/0003-066X.60.5.410

Sheldon, K. M., Boehm, J., & Lyubomirsky, S. (2013). Variety is the spice of happiness: The hedonic adaptation prevention model. In S. A. David, I. Boniwell, & A. Conley Ayers (Eds.), *The Oxford handbook of happiness* (pp. 901–914). Oxford University Press.

Sin, N. L., & Lyubomirsky, S. (2009). Enhancing well-being and alleviating depressive symptoms with positive psychology interventions: A practice-friendly meta-analysis. *Journal of Clinical Psychology*, 65(5), 467–487. https://doi-org.elib.tcd.ie/10.1002/jclp.20593

Swann, C., Carmona, C., Ryan, M., Baris, E., Dundson, S., & Kelly, M. P. (2010). Health systems and health-related behaviour change: A review of primary and secondary evidence. *National Institute for Health and Clinical Excellence*, 77.

WHO. (2021a). *Noncommunicable diseases*. www.who.int/news-room/fact-sheets/detail/noncommunicable-diseases

WHO. (2021b). *Suicide*. www.who.int/news-room/fact-sheets/detail/suicide

WHO. (2021c). *Basic documents*. https://apps.who.int/gb/bd/pdf_files/BD_49th-en.pdf#page=6

WHO. (2021d). *Diet and Physical Activity*. www.who.int/dietphysicalactivity/media/en/gsfs_general.pdf

Part II
Health and wellbeing tools

2 Calming tools

Introduction

When we think of positive emotions, we usually consider joy, happiness, excitement; in other words, emotions that are based on activation, which relates to doing or achieving something and to high energy. At the same time, emotions that help us soothe, feel content, safe, or peaceful are mentioned less frequently in the wellbeing literature (Gilbert, 2014). This chapter introduces a range of techniques that help us become calmer.

What does being calmer mean, and is it necessary? Most of us will agree that the phrase "everything in moderation" is a good motto to live by. It implies balance. The same can be said for how we manage *being* versus *doing*. Without *doing*, we would never have evolved as a species, never achieved anything, and never experienced the fullness of life in all its glory.

On the other hand, too much *doing* can lead to mental and physical distress and burnout (emotional and physical exhaustion), all of which can damage our relationships. Therefore, it makes sense that we should balance *doing* with *being*. Sometimes we need to slow down and appreciate life. *Being*, by its very nature, is calming and might be divided into (a) actions or activities that lead to a calm mind and body or (b) no action at all; mindfulness is a good example here, where we sit with eyes open or closed and watch everything that enters our awareness in a non-judgemental way.

Interestingly, our bodies (specifically our autonomic nervous system) can provide a concrete and practical way to balance *doing* with *being*. The autonomic nervous system (ANS) represents a collection of nerves that emerge from the brain and spinal column that control many bodily functions without the requirement for conscious control; we do not usually think about breathing, digesting food, or our heartbeat. The ANS is broken into two arms: the sympathetic and the parasympathetic systems. When we are in *doing* mode, the sympathetic ANS is in charge. Conversely, the parasympathetic is in charge when we are in *being* or calm mode.

It makes sense, then, that calming tools or activities activate the parasympathetic system. An example of this involves saliva production in the mouth. When we are in *doing* mode or when the sympathetic system is in overdrive (especially when we are anxious), our mouths become dry – saliva production stops. On the other hand, when we are calm and the parasympathetic system is in charge, saliva is often produced in the mouth. You can test this by overemphasising your exhalation when you breathe. When we inhale, we activate the sympathetic system, and when we exhale, we activate its counterpart. Try inhaling for 5 seconds, exhaling for 5 seconds, and then holding your breath for 5 seconds (all through your nose). Do this for a minute or two, and you will notice that saliva production in your mouth increases. This is *being* (calming) in action.

You will notice that many of the tools in this section involve those that require action or practice that encourage calm and those that require simply *being* (in nature or otherwise). There are many ways we can achieve calm in the mind and body; as always, it is essential to choose those that fit your temperament and lifestyle.

Calming tools include:

1 Sleep
2 Meditation
3 Nature
4 Creativity
5 Green care

Reference

Gilbert, P. (2014). The origins and nature of compassion focused therapy. *British Journal of Clinical Psychology*, *53*(1), 6–41. https://doi-org.elib.tcd.ie/10.1111/bjc.12043

Sleep

The World Health Organisation (WHO) recommends that people between 18 and 60 years achieve at least 7 hours of sleep each night (2004). However, approximately one-third of adults experience insomnia at any given time (Ohayon, 2011), which can harm our mental health. Interestingly, we tended to sleep more during the pandemic, and 42% of people abandoned their alarm clocks in the morning (Raman & Coogan,

2021), demonstrating the detrimental impact that the daily routine of getting ready for work can have on our sleep duration.

There are two types of insomnia, short-term and long-term (Frates et al., 2021). Short-term insomnia (lasting less than 3 months) can be caused by environmental factors (e.g. room temperature, lighting, noise), temporary pain due to physical illness, withdrawal of stimulants, e.g. coffee, or experiencing emotional distress. On the other hand, long-term (chronic) insomnia (occurring at least three times a week for over 3 months) is often caused by mental health issues or chronic physical illness. This is a two-way process whereby poor mental health can cause insomnia, and poor sleep can exacerbate mental health issues.

Furthermore, global rises in stress, poor stress management and burn-out among employees, and increased life-pressures caused by socioeconomic stressors contribute to poor sleep and insomnia (Salvagioni et al., 2017). Several interventions can help with insomnia and promote good sleep. These include cognitive behavioural therapy for insomnia, sleep hygiene education, physical exercise, yoga, mindfulness, weight loss, and light therapy (Takano et al., 2021). In this section, we will review additional research-based tools that can assist you in experiencing better-quality sleep.

Research-based tools

Tool 1: Breathing relaxation exercise (adapted from Wong et al., 2014)

Use a breathing phone app, e.g. The Breathing App (by Sergey Varichev, freely available in Google Play and App Store), to slow down your breathing for 30 minutes while lying in bed. If you don't want to use an app, you can do it yourself by counting your breaths. You aim to take five breaths per minute.

Tool 2: Maintain routine with children (adapted from Mindell et al., 2009)

If you have an infant or toddler at home, follow a three-step routine for the next 2 weeks to help them and you sleep better:

1. Bathe your child.
2. Massage them, or apply age-appropriate oil or moisturiser for older children.
3. Engage in quiet activities (e.g. cuddling, lullaby singing, book reading) and ensure that the lights are switched off within 30 minutes from the end of the bath.

Tool 3: Unplug (adapted from Hughes & Burke, 2018)

For the next 7 days, abstain from using your digital devices before going to bed. This includes your smartphone, computer, tablet, TV, etc. Leave them in another room or switch them off an hour or so before sleep. Finding alternative ways to spend your time without your phone is the last thing you will experience before falling asleep.

Tool 4: Listen to music (adapted from Pan & Pan, 2021)

Every night, before going to bed, listen to music for at least 10 minutes for the next week. It can be any type of music, such as music from various cultures (e.g. Chinese, Buddhist, Indian, Turkish), lullaby, new age, pop, classical, jazz, or others. If you wish to extend the positive effect of music, listen to it upon waking up as well.

Tool 5: Acupressure (adapted from Chen et al., 2020)

Acupressure is an alternative treatment method whereby pressure is applied to specific acupoints around the body. Learn about the sleep-related acupoints that you need to apply pressure to and do it before going to bed to improve your sleep quality.

Tool 6: Exercise (adapted from Lederman et al., 2019)

Engage in all forms of exercise (e.g. aerobic, tai chi, yoga, resistance training) throughout the day to help you sleep at night. Studies have shown that following a bog-standard exercise programme was more effective for sleep quality than individualising it to your preference.

Tool 7: Read a book before going to bed (Finucane et al., 2021)

For the next 7 days, read a book before going to bed, and the next day, reflect on the differences in your sleep quality. Please note it is better to read a printed book, as a digital book makes us less sleepy and delays sleep by 30 minutes (Grønli et al., 2016).

Tool 8: Night workers' sleep (McKenna & Wilkes, 2018)

Here are some of the research-based tools applied for those whose circadian rhythm is disturbed due to working at night:

- Pre-shift nap: nap between 2 and 6 p.m. for 60 to 90 minutes and follow it with caffeine
- Avoid caffeine at least 3 hours before you anticipate sleeping.

- Eat your main meal before the night shift and then a small meal during the night to prevent hunger.
- Avoid bright daylight when you go home after your shift. You can do it by wearing dark sunglasses.
- Apart from these night worker–specific tips, please use all other techniques mentioned in this book.

Variations of practice

Incorporate at least one of the calming tools in this book into your pre-bedtime plan. Other tools you may consider are:

- Have the same daily bed and wake-up times (including the weekend).
- Install blackout blinds.
- Reduce noise exposure with earplugs if necessary.
- Reduce smoking, and have your last caffeine-containing beverage in the afternoon.
- Reduce alcohol intake. Even though sometimes it helps us fall asleep, it affects our sleep quality.
- Reduce the temperature in your bedroom compared to the rest of your home.
- Start preparing for bed at 9 p.m. if you can.
- Try to have your last meal by 7 p.m. However, emerging research is inconclusive about this common belief and shows that eating 1 hour before sleep may be enough to have a good-quality sleep (Duan et al., 2021).
- Do your best to have a comfortable and tranquil bedroom.

Additional tools include (Frates et al., 2021):

- Dim your lights 1 or 2 hours before going to sleep.
- Take a warm bath or shower before going to bed.
- In order to get your circadian rhythm synchronised, make sure that you go outside and experience the daylight in the morning. If the first time you go outside is the afternoon, it may result in disturbed sleep at night.
- Keep your bedroom for sleep and sex only. Do not work there.
- Limit your nap throughout the day to 30 minutes.

Check out other tools in this book

Expressive writing has shown benefits for distressed people whose thoughts keep them awake at night (Arigo & Smyth, 2012). Also, mindfulness and meditation are effective at helping with sleep (Black et al., 2015). Finally, bibliotherapy using self-help books for insomnia is yet another useful technique to improve sleep length and quality. Gratitude can also improve your sleep quality (Jackowska et al., 2016).

Mental and physical health benefits

Our mental, physical, social, and environmental health are all integrated and dependent on each other. Therefore, poor psychology and social health will have a knock-on effect on the body and vice versa. The same is true for sleep. It is clear from the scientific literature that scientists have found it challenging to show that sleep has direct, causal positive impacts on specific aspects of our biology and psychology. Much of the research on the benefit of sleep among humans is observed indirectly from studying insomnia or disturbed sleep. Nevertheless, sleep is good for us and essential for living a good life.

A meta-analysis of studies assessing the impact of acupressure on the sleep quality of elderly adults showed that they were highly influential in improving participants' sleep quality and cognitive functioning (Chen et al., 2020). Exercise is beneficial for people with mental health issues who experience insomnia (Lederman et al., 2019). Alternative medicine interventions such as aromatherapy prove very effective in reducing insomnia and enhancing sleep quality, even more effective than massage (Hwang et al., 2015).

Sleep is particularly challenging for new parents. However, setting up a sleep routine promotes parents' and children's sleep quality (Mindell et al., 2009). Furthermore, it significantly reduces problematic sleep behaviours in children and the number of wakings throughout the night. At the same time, parental mood improves when they have the time to get a good night's sleep. The excellent news is that mood improves rapidly only three nights after implementing changes (Mindell et al., 2017); hence, it is worthwhile trying.

Using digital devices in bed before falling asleep has a negative impact on sleep quality, which is particularly risky for younger people (Bartel et al., 2014). In addition, increasing mobile use is associated with increased fatigue, shorter sleep, and later rise in the morning (Exelmans & Van den Bulck, 2016). In contrast, restricting the use of a smartphone for a week in the last hour before going to sleep was associated with increases in subjective wellbeing and quality of life and a decrease of smartphone addiction (Hughes & Burke, 2018).

Nightly sleep reduces the activity of many immune cells and the chemical messengers they produce (cytokines), while the converse is also true; long-term sleep disturbances can lead to an increase in inflammation, which is especially the case for those suffering from chronic inflammatory-related and cardiovascular diseases (Besedovsky et al., 2019). Unsurprisingly, poor sleep is a potent risk factor for developing high blood pressure, heart disease, and type 2 diabetes (Nagai et al., 2010). Therefore, it makes sense that adequate sleep will, in part (along with other healthy lifestyle changes like healthy diet and exercise), protect you from heart disease and diabetes.

Scientists have shown that we become more pessimistic when we do not get enough sleep; we experience a temporary drop in life satisfaction (Shin & Kim, 2018). On the other hand, adequate sleep has increased psychological resilience and life satisfaction (Shin & Kim, 2018). Adequate sleep reduces depression, anxiety, and stress; however, the evidence is less clear for conditions like post-traumatic stress disorder (PTSD), psychosis, burnout, rumination, and suicidal thinking (Scott et al., 2021). Few researchers have demonstrated successfully that sleep can improve attributes of positive psychology such as positive emotion, engagement, relationships, meaning, and accomplishment directly. Predictably, adequate sleep can indirectly help with relationships. For example, in a study of 42 American heterosexual couples, reduced sleep (less than 7 hours each night) led to increased negative behaviour during conflict (Wilson et al., 2017). Interestingly, couples who applied a positive behavioural approach that included practising humour, acceptance, acknowledgement (e.g. I can see that you are exhausted), self-disclosure (e.g. I am angry because I am tired), and constructive problem-solving managed to counteract these negative impacts (Wilson et al., 2017). Thus, sleep is good for connecting with others.

Caveat

Some disease processes can cause insomnia and sleep disturbances. It is vital to meet with your general practitioner or healthcare provider first to rule out any physical causes. Sleeping too much is not suitable for us either and can increase the risk of diabetes, heart disease, and earlier death. Exercising can help you improve your sleep quality and duration, but try to avoid exercising immediately before going to bed, as higher levels of adrenaline may prevent you from falling asleep.

References

Arigo, D., & Smyth, J. M. (2012). The benefits of expressive writing on sleep difficulty and appearance concerns for college women. *Psychology & Health*, *27*(2), 210–226. https://doi.org/10.1080/08870446.2011.558196

Bartel, K. A., Gradisar, M., & Williamson, P. (2015). Protective and risk factors for adolescent sleep: A meta-analytic review. *Sleep Medicine Reviews*, *21*, 72–85. https://doi-org.elib.tcd.ie/10.1016/j.smrv.2014.08.002

Besedovsky, L., Lange, T., & Haack, M. (2019). The sleep-immune crosstalk in health and disease. *Physiological Reviews*, *99*(3), 1325–1380. doi:10.1152/physrev.00010.2018

Black, D. S., O'Reilly, G. A., Olmstead, R., Breen, E. C., & Irwin, M. R. (2015). Mindfulness meditation and improvement in sleep quality and daytime impairment among older adults with sleep disturbances: A randomized clinical trial. *JAMA Internal Medicine*, *175*(4), 494–501. doi:10.1001/jamainternmed.2014.8081

Chen, M.-C., Yang, L.-Y., Chen, K.-M., & Hsu, H.-F. (2020). Systematic review and meta-analysis on using acupressure to promote the health of older adults. *Journal of Applied Gerontology*, *39*(10), 1144–1152. https://doi-org.elib.tcd.ie/10.1177/0733464819870027

Duan, D., Gu, C., Polotsky, V. Y., Jun, J. C., & Pham, L. V. (2021). Effects of dinner timing on sleep stage distribution and EEG power spectrum in healthy volunteers. *National Science of Sleep*, *13*, 601–612. https://doi.org/10.2147/NSS.S301113

Exelmans, L., & Van den Bulck, J. (2016). Bedtime mobile phone use and sleep in adults. *Social Science & Medicine (1982)*, *148*, 93–101. https://doi.org/10.1016/j.socscimed.2015.11.037

Finucane, E., O'Brien, A., Treweek, S., Newell, J., Das, K., Chapman, S., Wicks, P., Galvin, S., Healy, P., Biesty, L., Gillies, K., Noel-Storr, A., Gardner, H., O'Reilly, M. F., & Devane, D. (2021). Does reading a book in bed make a difference to sleep in comparison to not reading a book in bed? The people's trial-an online, pragmatic, randomised trial. *Trials*, *22*(1), 873. https://doi-org.elib.tcd.ie/10.1186/s13063-021-05831-3

Frates, B., Bonnet, J. P., Joseph, R., & Peterson, M. A. (2021). *Lifestyle medicine handbook: An introduction to the power of healthy habits* (2nd ed.). Healthy Learning.

Grønli, J., Byrkjedal, I. K., Bjorvatn, B., Nødtvedt, Ø., Hamre, B., & Pallesen, S. (2016). Reading from an iPad or from a book in bed: The impact on human sleep. A randomized controlled crossover trial. *Sleep Medicine*, *21*, 86–92. https://doi-org.elib.tcd.ie/10.1016/j.sleep.2016.02.006

Hughes, N., & Burke, J. (2018). Sleeping with the frenemy: How restricting 'bedroom use' of smartphones impacts happiness and wellbeing. *Computers in Human Behavior*, *85*, 236–244. https://doi-org.elib.tcd.ie/10.1016/j.chb.2018.03.047

Hwang, E., & Shin, S. (2015). The effects of aromatherapy on sleep improvement: A systematic literature review and meta-analysis. *Journal of Alternative & Complementary Medicine*, *21*(2), 61–68. https://doi-org.elib.tcd.ie/10.1089/acm.2014.0113

Jackowska, M., Brown, J., Ronaldson, A., & Steptoe, A. (2016). The impact of a brief gratitude intervention on subjective wellbeing, biology and sleep. *Journal of Health Psychology*, *21*(10), 2207–2217. https://doi.org/10.1177/1359105315572455

Lederman, O., Ward, P. B., Firth, J., Maloney, C., Carney, R., Vancampfort, D., Stubbs, B., Kalucy, M., & Rosenbaum, S. (2019). Does exercise improve sleep quality in individuals with mental illness? A systematic review and meta-analysis.

Journal of Psychiatric Research, 109, 96–106. https://doi-org.elib.tcd.ie/10.1016/j.jpsychires.2018.11.004

McKenna, H., & Wilkes, M. (2018). Optimising sleep for night shifts. BMJ (Clinical Research Ed.), 360, j5637. https://doi-org.elib.tcd.ie/10.1136/bmj.j5637

Mindell, J. A., Leichman, E. S., Lee, C., Williamson, A. A., & Walters, R. M. (2017). Implementation of a nightly bedtime routine: How quickly do things improve? Infant Behavior & Development, 49, 220–227. https://doi-org.elib.tcd.ie/10.1016/j.infbeh.2017.09.013

Mindell, J. A., Telofski, L. S., Wiegand, B., & Kurtz, E. S. (2009). A nightly bedtime routine: Impact on sleep in young children and maternal mood. Sleep, 32(5), 599–606. https://doi.org/10.1093/sleep/32.5.599

Nagai, M., Hoshide, S., & Kario, K. (2010). Sleep duration as a risk factor for cardiovascular disease- a review of the recent literature. Current Cardiology Reviews, 6(1), 54–61. doi:10.2174/157340310790231635

Ohayon, M. M. (2011). Epidemiological overview of sleep disorders in the general population. Sleep Medicine Research, 2(1), 1–9. doi:10.17241/smr.2011.2.1.1

Pan, B-Y., & Pan, E. M. (2021). Can music improve sleep quality? A systematic literature review. Canadian Journal of Music Therapy, 27, 49–78.

Raman, S., & Coogan, A. N. (2021). Effects of societal-level COVID-19 mitigation measures on the timing and quality of sleep in Ireland. Sleep Medicine. https://doi-org.elib.tcd.ie/10.1016/j.sleep.2021.02.024

Salvagioni, D. A. J., Melanda, F. N., Mesas, A. E., González, A. D., Gabani, F. L., & Andrade, S. M. D. (2017). Physical, psychological and occupational consequences of job burnout: A systematic review of prospective studies. PLoS One, 12(10), e0185781–e0185781. doi:10.1371/journal.pone.0185781

Scott, A. J., Webb, T. L., Martyn-St James, M., Rowse, G., & Weich, S. (2021). Improving sleep quality leads to better mental health: A meta-analysis of randomised controlled trials. Sleep Medicine Reviews, 60, 101556. https://doi.org/10.1016/j.smrv.2021.101556

Shin, J.-E., & Kim, J. K. (2018). How a good sleep predicts life satisfaction: The role of zero-sum beliefs about happiness. Frontiers in Psychology, 9(1589). doi:10.3389/fpsyg.2018.01589

Takano, Y., Iwano, S., Aoki, S., Nakano, N., & Sakano, Y. (2021). A systematic review of the effect of sleep interventions on presenteeism. BioPsychoSocial Medicine, 15(1), 21. doi:10.1186/s13030-021-00224-z

WHO. (2004, January 22–24). WHO technical meeting on sleep and health. WHO.

Wilson, S. J., Jaremka, L. M., Fagundes, C. P., Andridge, R., Peng, J., Malarkey, W. B., . . . Kiecolt-Glaser, J. K. (2017). Shortened sleep fuels inflammatory responses to marital conflict: Emotion regulation matters. Psychoneuroendocrinology, 79, 74–83. doi:10.1016/j.psyneuen.2017.02.015

Wong, E. M.-L., Chair, S.-Y., Leung, D. Y., & Chan, S. W.-C. (2014). Can a brief educational intervention improve sleep and anxiety outcomes for emergency orthopaedic surgical patients? Contemporary Nurse: A Journal for the Australian Nursing Profession, 47(1/2), 132–143. https://search.informit.org/doi/10.3316/informit.796159412060574

Meditation

The Roman emperor and philosopher Marcus Aurelius stated that the happiness of life depends upon the quality of an individual's thoughts. Many of the problems we face as human beings originate in thought and how we perceive the world around us. These problems can manifest as anxiety, loss of focus and attention, emotional regulation problems, psychosomatic symptoms related to gut health, tension headaches, and fatigue. Meditation practice can be part of the solution here, not just for mitigating symptoms but also for promoting flourishing and wellbeing. Although many believe that meditation is about stopping thinking to achieve an empty mind (a state when you do not think about anything), the reality remains that it is not possible to eradicate these mental and physical processes. Instead, many meditation practices are concerned with disengaging from thoughts, memories, emotions, and sensations on a moment-by-moment basis and in a non-judgemental way. The simple but powerful practice of sitting still and upright with eyes closed for minutes at a time can exert enormous benefits on our psychosocial and physical health, benefits that have been documented by research scientists across the world (Gawrylewski, 2018).

Research-based tools

We can break meditation into three basic practices that have different impacts on the mind and body (Singer & Engert, 2019). Meditation practices usually involve sitting gently upright with eyes closed. However, many variations exist that include (1) concentration-based mediations which focus on a chosen phrase (mantra) or the breath, (2) awareness-based meditations (mindfulness), and (3) those practices that cultivate compassion (loving-kindness meditation). Many religions and belief structures such as Buddhism and Hinduism incorporate all three types of meditation in their daily practice. In this section, we will include only selected practices. However, evidence exists for many different types of meditation.

Tool 9: Mindfulness – body scan (Kabat-Zinn, 1990)

Mindfulness practice cultivates awareness of body and mind. The goal is to observe and accept thoughts, emotions, sensations, and memories on a moment-by-moment basis in a non-judgemental way. You can extend mindfulness practice to involve activities conducted with eyes open, including mindful eating, walking, cooking, and creative pursuits. The

Body Scan is an excellent example of mindful practice that focuses specifically on the body. There are many online guided versions of the Body Scan that vary in length, languages, accents, and voice. Thus, the most suitable version of Body Scan can be used.

To practice on your own, begin by adopting a comfortable posture (lying down if you prefer). Breathe normally and bring your attention to the toes of your left foot. Slowly and gently, bring your attention up through your left leg, across your pelvis, and down to the toes of your right foot. Repeat the process with your right leg. Next, move to the base of your back and move up either side of your spine before resting at your shoulders. Move down to the tips of the fingers in both hands and back up through your arms. From your shoulders, move to the back of your neck, around to your throat, jaw, and face. Relax your eye muscles before moving up to your scalp. Finish by taking a low, slow, and deep breath in through your nose, followed by a gentle exhalation, also through your nose. The Body Scan can be as long or short as you like.

Tool 10: Concentration-based meditation (Dunne et al., 2019)

This meditation practice employs an anchor such as the breath or a chosen phrase (mantra) to develop a focus and attention that *transcend* (but do not stop) turbulent thought, emotion, memories, and physical sensations. The aim is to disengage without interaction of any kind with mental and physical processes. Examples include attention-based training (ABT: Dunne et al., 2019), mantra, and Zazen (Japanese) sitting meditation (Suzuki & Dixon, 2020), among others. Each time the practitioner is distracted by thoughts, emotions, or sensations, they gently return to their chosen anchor, which can be the breath or a mantra. This type of meditation can also be practised with eyes open, focusing on an external object (e.g. candle, image, bright phone screen).

ABT can be practised as follows:

- Sit in a gentle upright position; feet on the floor, hands on your lap.
- Set a timer for 2 minutes.
- If possible, close your eyes; if you don't want to close your eyes, you can pick a focal point in front of you, such as a picture on the wall.
- Focus on your breathing process or a mantra ("I am here now").
- Remember to breathe normally throughout.
- Each time you become distracted by memories, thoughts, sensations, and emotions, disengage and return to your anchor.
- When your timer goes off, open your eyes and enjoy the feeling of being present.

Begin your practice with 2 minutes twice daily for the first 2 weeks. After that, go at your own pace; be gentle with yourself. If you can, add 1 minute each week until you reach 10 minutes of practice at least once daily.

Tool 11: Meditation focused on cultivating compassion and gratitude
(Lama, 2012)

This practice category demonstrates how meditation can be used as a specific tool for cultivating particular behaviour. For example, in loving-kindness meditation, the practitioner uses specific imagery to cultivate compassion for self and others. You can also cultivate gratitude through a meditation using the essential practice (sitting upright and silent with eyes closed) to provide the foundation for compiling reasons to be grateful. For example, for loving-kindness meditation, use the mantra "I wish you health and happiness". Extend this wish to the focus of your attention, which might also include yourself.

Variations of practice

Meditation practices vary significantly. Variations include guided meditations that employ imagery and/or music, group or community practice, chanting, and certain types of prayer. Focused breathing is important in most meditation practices. For some, the breath is used as a foundation for practice (concentration-based meditation). In contrast, other practices use specific types of breathing that can involve varying emphases on the duration and depth of inhalation and exhalation cycles.

Check out other tools in this book

Nature tools induce mindfulness as well and are worthwhile exploring.

Mental and physical health benefits

Meditation practises are very useful for relationship enhancement. For example, eight weekly sessions and a full-day retreat resulted in increases in couples' satisfaction with the relationship, closeness, acceptance of partner, relaxation, optimism, not to mention higher levels of spirituality and decline in psychological and relationship distress (Carson et al., 2004). Furthermore, in a 6-year follow up of a once-off mindfulness programme lasting 7 weeks with 2-hour sessions twice a week and two booster sessions every year for 6 years, participants reported higher levels of wellbeing; they used more effective coping strategies when facing adversity. The good news is that even self-administered, short-term online mindfulness can boost a range of positive outcomes. For example, an 8-week programme during which participants were asked to listen to a mindfulness audio 12 minutes a day and an 8- to 10-minute introduction video resulted in increased hedonic, eudaimonic wellbeing, compassion for others and self-compassion, gratitude, and other positive outcomes (Ivtzan et al., 2016). Meditation practice positively impacts mental health (Keng et al., 2011). It is particularly useful for reducing anxiety, stress, and burnout (Dunne et al., 2019) and improving sleep quality, latency, and duration (Black et al., 2015; Shallcross et al., 2019). Sleep has a positive impact on the immune (David S. Black & Slavich, 2016) and cardiovascular systems (Levine et al., 2017), as well as on brain structure and function (Ricard et al., 2014). Meditation modifies brain activity, allowing for greater focus, attention, and cognitive control as well as emotional regulation (Tang et al., 2015). Initial studies also indicate that meditation practices might help practitioners manage discomfort caused by chronic disease states (Ridge et al., 2021; Victorson et al., 2015).

Caveat

Individuals suffering from trauma (past or current) are advised not to engage in meditation without professional support. Meditation can sometimes accentuate trauma-related imagery and expose the individual to disturbing memories or thought processes. Likewise, those experiencing recent grief are cautioned not to practice loving-kindness meditation, which might lead to upset; loving-kindness meditation places a strong emphasis on cultivating mental images of those we love. Individuals with active obsessive-compulsive thinking are advised to engage in meditation with caution and with the support of their healthcare provider. Sometimes we are not ready to meditate. It might be necessary for those experiencing anxiety, stress, or depression to engage in practices that cultivate physical activity in a safe setting before meditation-based practices. Meditation is complex and can take a significant amount of time to master, especially if one has a highly active mind or frequently uses external distractions to manage stress or anxiety.

References

Black, D. S., O'Reilly, G. A., Olmstead, R., Breen, E. C., & Irwin, M. R. (2015). Mindfulness meditation and improvement in sleep quality and daytime impairment among older adults with sleep disturbances: A randomized clinical trial. *JAMA Internal Medicine*, *175*(4), 494–501. doi:10.1001/jamainternmed.2014.8081

Black, D. S., & Slavich, G. M. (2016). Mindfulness meditation and the immune system: A systematic review of randomized controlled trials. *Annals of the New York Academy of Sciences, 1373*(1), 13–24. doi:10.1111/nyas.12998

Carson, J. W., Carson, K. M., Gil, K. M., & Baucom, D. H. (2004). Mindfulness-based relationship enhancement. *Behavioural Therapy, 35,* 471–494.

de Vibe, M., Solhaug, I., Rosenvinge, J. H., Tyssen, R., Hanley, A., & Garland, E. (2018). Six-year positive effects of a mindfulness-based intervention on mindfulness, coping and wellbeing in medical and psychology students: Results from a randomized controlled trial. *PLoS One, 13,* e0196053.

Dunne, P. J., Lynch, J., Prihodova, L., O'Leary, C., Ghoreyshi, A., Basdeo, S. A., . . . White, B. (2019). Burnout in the emergency department: Randomized controlled trial of an attention-based training program. *Journal of Integrative Medicine, 17*(3), 173–180. https://doi.org/10.1016/j.joim.2019.03.009

Gawrylewski, A. (2018). Be a better you (smart, happy, relaxed). *Scientific American Mind, 27,* 1–112.

Ivtzan, I., Young, T., Martman, J., Jeffrey, A., Lomas, T., Hart, R., & Eiroa-Orosa, F. J. (2016). Integrating mindfulness into positive psychology: A randomised controlled trial of an online positive mindfulness program. *Mindfulness, 7*(6), 1396–1407. https://doi-org.elib.tcd.ie/10.1007/s12671-016-0581-1

Kabat-Zinn, J. (1990). *Full catastrophe living: Using the wisdom of your body and mind to face stress, pain and illness* (1st ed.). Delta.

Keng, S. L., Smoski, M. J., & Robins, C. J. (2011). Effects of mindfulness on psychological health: A review of empirical studies. *Clinical Psychology Review, 31*(6), 1041–1056. doi:10.1016/j.cpr.2011.04.006

Lama, D. (2012). *How to be compassionate: A handbook for creating inner peace and a happier world.* Ebury Publishing.

Levine, G. N., Lange, R. A., Bairey-Merz, C. N., Davidson, R. J., Jamerson, K., Mehta, P. K., . . . Smith, S. C., Jr. (2017). Meditation and cardiovascular risk reduction: A scientific statement from the American heart association. *Journal of the American Heart Association, 6*(10). doi:10.1161/jaha.117.002218

Ricard, M., Lutz, A., & Davidson, R. J. (2014). Mind of the meditator. *Scientific American, 311*(5), 38–45. doi:10.1038/scientificamerican1114-38

Ridge, K., Conlon, N., Hennessy, M., & Dunne, P. J. (2021). Feasibility assessment of an 8-week attention-based training programme in the management of chronic spontaneous urticaria. *Pilot and Feasibility Studies, 7*(1), 103. doi:10.1186/s40814-021-00841-z

Shallcross, A. J., Visvanathan, P. D., Sperber, S. H., & Duberstein, Z. T. (2019). Waking up to the problem of sleep: Can mindfulness help? A review of theory and evidence for the effects of mindfulness for sleep. *Current Opinion in Psychology, 28,* 37–41. https://doi.org/10.1016/j.copsyc.2018.10.005

Singer, T., & Engert, V. (2019). It matters what you practice: Differential training effects on subjective experience, behavior, brain and body in the resource project. *Current Opinion in Psychology, 28,* 151–158. https://doi.org/10.1016/j.copsyc.2018.12.005

Suzuki, S., & Dixon, T. (2020). *Zen mind, beginner's mind: 50th Anniversary Edition.* Shambhala.

Tang, Y. Y., Hölzel, B. K., & Posner, M. I. (2015). The neuroscience of mindfulness meditation. *Nature Reviews Neuroscience*, *16*(4), 213–225. doi:10.1038/nrn3916

Victorson, D., Kentor, M., Maletich, C., Lawton, R. C., Kaufman, V. H., Borrero, M., . . . Berkowitz, C. (2015). Mindfulness meditation to promote wellness and manage chronic disease: A systematic review and meta-analysis of mindfulness-based randomized controlled trials relevant to lifestyle medicine. *American Journal of Lifestyle Medicine*, *9*(3), 185–211. doi:10.1177/1559827614537789

Nature

Spending time in nature can often be a challenge, especially if you live in an urban area. Yet at the same time, it is one of the sources of calm, awe, and serenity. As a wellbeing tool, nature can be perceived from two perspectives: (1) nature contact and (2) nature connectedness. Nature contact means that we interact with nature on an ad-hoc or more regular basis by going for walks or reviewing photographs or art associated with trees, flowers, and other natural environments. Alternatively, we surround ourselves with plants, herbs, growing vegetables and flowers. Nature connectedness refers to the personal connection we feel with nature, for example, being moved by the beauty of a lark singing or watching the fog dawdling through the valley. Some of us are more sensitive to nature than others and profoundly connect with it. The good news is that nature interventions are even more effective for those who find it challenging to connect with nature (Richardson et al., 2019), so why not give it a try?

Research-based tools

Tool 12: Visit nature (adapted from Martin et al., 2020; Nisbet, 2014)

Whether you live in the countryside or an urban area, go outside for at least half an hour once a week. It doesn't matter what you do when outside. You may go for a walk, sit on a bench basking in the sun or play ball with your children. What matters is that you are outside.

Tool 13: Three good things in nature (adapted from Keenan et al., 2021)

If you live in a rural area, go for a walk to a forest, park, beach, mountain, lakeside, or bog area for half an hour every day for 5 consecutive days. If you live in an urban area, go through a housing estate, town centre, town park, or main road. Try to vary your walk each day. Also, you can go on your own or with another person or a group of people. It is up to you; however, this tool was assessed as a group activity. As you walk each day, try to notice three good things in nature. Then, when you are in the company of others, share the three things that you noticed.

Tool 14: Imagine yourself in nature (adapted from Ryan et al., 2010)

If you don't have access to nature but want to avail yourself of the benefits associated with it, close your eyes and imagine yourself being in nature. Picture a specific place, be it a beach or a forest, a road, or your favourite market square. Imagine you are there right now; feel the wind on your skin, the sun burning your face, or the raindrops on your head. The more effort you put into visualising it, the greater your result.

Tool 15: The sound of nature (adapted from Luo et al., 2021)

Search for a phone application or web recording of the sound of nature. Play it in the background for 30 minutes each day while you complete a task, especially one that requires your cognitive skills. Repeat this activity for as many days as you wish. Researchers asked participants to do it every day for 4 weeks and found that it promoted health and wellbeing.

Tool 16: Noticing nature (adapted from Passmore & Holder, 2016)

Over the next 2 weeks, become mindful of how nature made you feel. When any place or object evokes powerful emotion in you, take a picture and share it on your social media or via instant messaging with a description of an emotion you've experienced. In the original study, participants shared approximately ten photographs over 2 weeks and uploaded them to a researchers' folder, not social media.

Variations of practice

It is essential to be picky when selecting nature walks, because higher-quality nature settings are associated with a more significant psychological impact (Wyles et al., 2019). Therefore, go the extra mile to a natural place you consider worth visiting. Each year, David Suzuki's Foundation's 30x30 Nature Challenge encourages Canadians to spend 30 minutes every day in May outside in nature, which results in a great mood and vitality improvements (Nisbet, 2014), so if committing to daily walks is too much for you, try to do it for a limited amount of time, be it a week or a month. Invite your friends to do it with you to gain more benefits from the nature connection. If you are a coach or a therapist, consider walk-and-talk therapy instead of sitting indoors with your clients, as it can enrich your practice (Revell & McLeod, 2017). Another activity, which is a twist on the Sound of Nature, is the Savouring Nature tool (Steidle et al., 2017):

- Listen to a nature soundscape (e.g. birdsong, sea sounds, forest trees in the wind).
- Ground yourself with 1 minute of focusing on your breath.
- Use your senses and imagination to imagine yourself in the natural setting of the soundscape.
- Immerse yourself in the experience fully for 5 minutes.
- To end the exercise, start to move your fingers and focus on your breath as you slowly open your eyes and come back into the room for 1 minute.

Check out other tools in this book

The Photography Tools involve nature; it may be beneficial to combine them. Also, the Blue Spaces Tool provides additional ideas on how to spend time in nature.

Mental and physical health benefits

More than 238 outdoor nature and adventure tourists were recently interviewed and asked whether they are happy and therefore chose to visit nature or whether it is nature that makes them happy (Buckley, 2020). More than 80% responded that being in nature made them happy. Furthermore, almost 90% claimed short-term benefits, and 60% reported that nature helped them cope with stress more effectively. In a sample of more than 6,000 women, the researchers found that many found refuge in nature from the psychological trauma they experienced (Buckley & Westaway, 2021).

Spending at least 120 minutes a week in nature is associated with improved self-reported physical health and enhanced levels of wellbeing (White et al., 2019). These 2 hours in nature can be experienced as one long or short visits a week. Moreover, feeling connected with nature results in higher levels of happiness and deeper (eudaimonic) wellbeing; visiting nature at least once a week is associated with good physical health (Capaldi et al., 2014; Martin et al., 2020). When we feel connected with nature, our psychological resilience grows (Ingulli & Lindbloom, 2013), and we feel more intrinsically motivated to engage in daily activities.

Walking in nature, as opposed to walking indoors, is associated with higher levels of vitality (Ryan et al., 2010). Thus it is the nature rather than physical activity that makes a difference. An intervention which compared noticing the *beauty of nature* versus *human-built areas* showed that those who spent time in nature experienced more elevating experiences and a general sense of connectedness to nature, people, and life as a whole (Passmore & Holder, 2016). In addition to helping people feel well, nature walks also reduce symptoms of depression and anxiety (Keenan et al., 2021), sadness, anger, and fatigue (Bowler et al., 2010). A systematic review of the benefits of outdoor walking groups identified a significant reduction in participants' systolic blood pressure, diastolic blood pressure, resting heart rate, body fat, body mass index, and total cholesterol (Hanson & Jones, 2015). However, it is impossible to determine if the change was in nature or the walking group's physical activity.

To enjoy the benefits of nature, we don't need to go outside. When compared with listening to classical music or enjoying the silence, those who listen to the sound of nature report a significant reduction in muscle tension, pulse rate, and self-reported stress (Largo-Wight et al., 2016). Furthermore, a 4-week intervention of listening daily to the sounds of nature significantly improved the experience of positive emotions and improved cognitive performance, i.e. attention, experiences of flow, and working memory (Luo et al., 2021). Thus, being in nature offers a range of physiological and psychological benefits.

A large-scale research study with cancer patients identified that nature was one of the most important resources for them when coping with illness (Ahmadi & Ahmadi, 2015). In particular, listening to nature and engaging in any activity outdoors was perceived as a spiritual journey that helped them feel significantly better. The benefit of being in nature for both clinical and non-clinical populations may be due to the fact that when in nature, repetitive negative thoughts are reduced as the subgenual prefrontal cortex of our brain is activated, which his responsible for regulating our emotions and giving us a feeling of reward (Bratman et al., 2015). Being in nature is like winning a prize over and over again.

Caveat

When connecting with nature, practice caution and safety first. Avoid secluded or dangerous places. Join walking groups or try to arrange spending time in nature with others. Let your friends and family know where you are going before you leave your home.

References

Ahmadi, F., & Ahmadi, N. (2015). Nature as the most important coping strategy among cancer patients: A Swedish Survey. *Journal of Religion and Health*, 54(4), 1177–1190. https://doi-org.elib.tcd.ie/10.1007/s10943-013-9810-2

Bowler, D. E., Buyung-Ali, L. M., Knight, T. M., & Pullin, A. S. (2010). A systematic review of evidence for the added benefits to health of exposure to natural environments. *BMC Public Health*, *10*(1), 456–465. https://doi-org.elib.tcd.ie/10.1186/1471-2458-10-456

Bratman, G. N., Hamilton, J. P., Hahn, K. S., Daily, G. C., & Gross, J. J. (2015). Nature experience reduces rumination and subgenual prefrontal cortex activation. *PNAS Proceedings of the National Academy of Sciences of the United States of America*, *112*(28), 8567–8572. https://doi-org.elib.tcd.ie/10.1073/pnas.1510459112

Buckley, R. (2020). Nature tourism and mental health: Parks, happiness, and causation. *Journal of Sustainable Tourism*, *28*(9), 1409–1424. doi:10.1080/09669582.2020.1742725

Buckley, R., & Westaway, D. (2021). Women report that nature tourism provides recovery from psychological trauma. *Tourism Recreation Research*. doi:10.1080/02508281.2021.1917892

Capaldi, C. A., Dopko, R. L., & Zelenski, J. M. (2014). The relationship between nature connectedness and happiness: A meta-analysis. *Frontiers in Psychology*, *5*, 976. https://doi.org/10.3389/fpsyg.2014.00976

Hanson, S., & Jones, A. (2015). Is there evidence that walking groups have health benefits? A systematic review and meta-analysis. *British Journal of Sports Medicine*, *49*(11), 710–715. https://doi-org.elib.tcd.ie/10.1136/bjsports-2014-094157

Ingulli, K., & Lindbloom, G. (2013). Connection to nature and psychological resilience. *Ecopsychology*, *5*(1), 52–55. https://doi.org/10.1089/eco.2012.0042

Keenan, R., Lumber, R., Richardson, M., & Sheffield, D. (2021). Three good things in nature: A nature-based positive psychological intervention to improve mood and wellbeing for depression and anxiety. *Journal of Public Mental Health*, *20*(4), 243–250. https://doi-org.elib.tcd.ie/10.1108/JPMH-02-2021-0029

Largo-Wight, E., O'Hara, B. K., & Chen, W. W. (2016). The efficacy of a brief nature sound intervention on muscle tension, pulse rate, and self-reported stress. *Health Environments Research & Design Journal (HERD)* (Sage Publications, Ltd.), *10*(1), 45–51. https://doi-org.elib.tcd.ie/10.1177/193758671561974

Luo, J., Wang, M., & Chen, L. (2021). The effects of using a nature-sound mobile application on psychological well-being and cognitive performance among university students. *Frontiers in Psychology*, *12*, 699908. https://doi-org.elib.tcd.ie/10.3389/fpsyg.2021.699908

Martin, L., White, M. P., Hunt, A., Richardson, M., Pahl, S., & Burt, J. (2020). Nature contact, nature connectedness and associations with health, wellbeing and pro-environmental behaviours. *Journal of Environmental Psychology*, *68*. https://doi-org.elib.tcd.ie/10.1016/j.jenvp.2020.101389

Nisbet, E. K. (2014). *Canadians connect with nature and increase their well-being: Results of the 2014 David Suzuki Foundation 30x30 nature challenge*. Trent University.

Passmore, H. A., & Holder, M. D. (2017). Noticing nature: Individual and social benefits of a two-week intervention. *The Journal of Positive Psychology*, *12*(6), 537–546. doi:10.1080/17439760.2016.1221126

Revell, S., & McLeod, J. (2017). Therapists' experience of walk and talk therapy: A descriptive phenomenological study. *European Journal of Psychotherapy & Counselling*, *19*(3), 267–289. https://doi-org.elib.tcd.ie/10.1080/13642537.2017.1348377

Richardson, M., Hunt, A., Hinds, J., Bragg, R., Fido, D., Petronzi, D., Barbett, L., Clitherow, T., & White, M. (2019). A measure of nature connectedness for children and adults: Validation, performance, and insights. *Sustainability, 11*, 3250. https://doi.org/10.3390/su11123250

Ryan, R. M., Weinstein, N., Bernstein, J., Brown, K. W., Mistretta, L., & Gagné, M. (2010). Vitalizing effects of being outdoors and in nature. *Journal of Environmental Psychology, 30*(2), 159–168. https://doi-org.elib.tcd.ie/10.1016/j.jenvp.2009.10.009

Steidle, A., Gonzalez-Morales, M. G., Hoppe, A., Michel, A., & O'shea, D. (2017). Energizing respites from work: A randomized controlled study on respite interventions. *European Journal of Work and Organizational Psychology, 26*(5), 650–662. https://doi-org.elib.tcd.ie/10.1080/1359432X.2017.1348348

White, M. P., Alcock, I., Grellier, J., Wheeler, B. W., Hartig, T., Warber, S. L., Bone, A., Depledge, M. H., & Fleming, L. E. (2019). Spending at least 120 minutes a week in nature is associated with good health and wellbeing. *Scientific Reports, 9*(1), 7730. https://doi-org.elib.tcd.ie/10.1038/s41598-019-44097-3

Wyles, K. J., White, M. P., Hattam, C., Pahl, S., King, H., & Austen, M. (2019). Are some natural environments more psychologically beneficial than others? The importance of type and quality on connectedness to nature and psychological restoration. *Environment and Behavior, 51*(2), 111–143. https://doi.org/10.1177/0013916517738312

Creativity

The concept of 10,000 hours has received a lot of attention, especially after Malcolm Gladwell's book *Blink*, in which he provided examples of some of the most successful people, such as the Beatles or Steve Jobs, who, by the time they reached the age of 20, had put in approximately 10,000 hours to master their skill. Gladwell argued that nurture matters more than nature, and as such, anyone who has an opportunity for long-term deep practice can achieve extraordinary results. However, there are at least four fundamental problems with this way of thinking: (1) some people acquire knowledge faster than others; (2) despite knowing, some people show more creativity than others; (3) there is a genetic predisposition towards creativity; and (4) creativity is associated with other characteristics, such as open-mindedness (Simonton, 2021). This is why seeing creativity as being partially related to nature and nurture is more helpful. Also, acknowledging that there are many different types of creativity can help us understand and appreciate all that is good about us.

According to Beghetto and Kaufman (2007), some people have big-C Creativity whereby they are creative in the traditional sense of the word and contribute exponentially to arts or science, e.g. Da Vinci, Einstein, Beyoncé. Others have little-c creativity, meaning that they are great at problem-solving in their daily lives. Consider anyone in your life who can help you find a solution to a problem you may have grappled with for a while. The chances are that they boast little-c creativity. Some people have pro-c creativity, whereby they display extraordinary creativity in a professional domain of their lives. For example, a computer programmer could develop extraordinary coding that helps the police find a culprit. Finally, some of us may have mini-c creativity, meaning that we have a natural capacity for self-discovery, self-analysis, and self-improvement. An example of such a person is Helen Keller, who lost her sight and hearing when she was 19 months old (1903) and whose insights about topics such as optimism have helped millions of people and prompted a stream of psychological research. Regardless of what type of creativity you have, practising it is instrumental in helping us experience higher levels of wellbeing.

Research-based tools

Tool 17: Improvisation (adapted from Schwenke et al., 2021)

Improvisation, often referred to as "improv", is a process of thinking on one's feet, whereby storytelling, dialogue, or characters are created spontaneously. You can practice it regularly at work, during meetings, with your children when playing, or with your friends when attending social occasions. Furthermore, you can join one of the improv groups (e.g. https://improwiki.com/en/list_of_improv_groups_worldwide), established worldwide, that allow you to practice improv on stage.

Tool 18: Art-lift (adapted from Crone et al., 2013)

Attend a creative arts course in your vicinity for approximately 10 weeks, e.g. ceramics, drawing, mosaic, painting, poetry.

Tool 19: Mood repair (adapted from Dalebroux et al., 2008)

After experiencing something negative (e.g. watching an upsetting programme on TV, having an argument, or experiencing a few hassles during the day), pull out a sheet of drawing paper, paint (e.g. oil, acrylics), and draw or paint a picture depicting happiness or other positive emotions (e.g. calm, serenity, awe, pride, contentment). There is no time limit to this activity, and hopefully, afterwards, you will experience more balanced emotions.

ations of practice

When it comes to doing something creative, let your imagination run wild. Using your strength of creativity in whatever area of creativity you excel in can be good for you. Recently, a survey was carried out with more than 8,000 participants who regularly engage in crocheting, which is a very creative activity (Burns & Van Der Meer, 2021). Most of them crocheted three or more times a week and compared this activity to mindfulness. The results showed that crocheting made them feel more creative, calmer, happier, and more valuable.

Furthermore, when they engaged in crocheting at least once a week, it improved their confidence levels, calmness, happiness, and feeling useful. Many mentioned a reduction in perceived pain they experienced as part of existing illness. The researchers are calling for turning crocheting into a wellbeing intervention. While more research is required about crocheting, knitting, and similar activities, in the meantime, you may give it a try and see if it works for you.

Check out other tools in this book

Extensive research, especially with children, suggests that play enhances creativity. Please check out the Play tools in this book. Also, given that improv such as storytelling impacts creativity, check out the Storytelling tool in an emerging tool section.

Mental and physical health benefits

Creativity tools come in two formats; some aim to improve creativity, which is seen as a positive outcome; others enhance wellbeing, which is an additional positive outcome of creativity development (Forgeard & Eichner, 2014). For example, creative improvisation boosts psychological wellbeing (Schwenke et al., 2021). Art therapy and art making are the most effective Creativity tools to enhance wellness. For example, attending a 10-week creative arts course organised by the general practice was associated with a significant increase in various aspects of wellbeing (Crone et al., 2013). In addition, engaging in a rapid art project, e.g. painting a picture, can lift your mood after experiencing adversity (Dalebroux et al., 2008). This is consistent with the Broaden and Build theory, according to which positive emotions "undo" the negative emotions (Fredrickson et al., 2000).

Important research by Chilton and Wilkinson (2009) describes the ways in which art making in the art therapy and positive psychology intersect. They argue that art making supports optimism and happiness by giving individuals the experiences of flow and mastery. Bolwerk et al. (2014) demonstrated that actively creating art for 2 hours a week over a 10-week period can also have a positive impact on resilience. They believe that the making of art improves interaction between brain regions involved in tasks that support resilience like self-reflection and self-awareness and even memory processing. Thus, the impact of creativity goes beyond wellbeing.

However, a link continues to exist between the "mad genius" perception of creativity and mental illness, whereby some of the most creative minds (e.g. Vincent van Gogh, Sylvia Plath, Amy Winehouse) experienced severe mental health issues whilst also displaying extraordinary creativity (Zhao et al., 2021). This link has mainly been challenged by research showing that those people were creative not because of their mental illness but despite it. There is no significant relationship between mental disorders and creativity (Paek et al., 2016). Furthermore, their most fertile period of creativity often happened when their mental health symptoms were at moderate levels, thus suggesting that creativity can soothe and help during distress, not that mental illness is necessary to induce creativity.

Incidentally, inconclusive results exist concerning the impact of stress on creativity. While some research suggests that creativity decreases with time pressure due to the depletion of cognitive resources, other research demonstrates that it may result in higher motivation for as long as the stress is moderate, thus differentiating between a *challenge* – positive impact – and a *threat* – negative impact (Akinola et al., 2019). Furthermore, in surprising research findings, creative problem-solving was linked with the cerebellum, which is also responsible for deep practice and practice-makes-perfect activities (Saggar et al., 2015), which may be why creativity has been linked with the 10,000 hours we mentioned earlier.

Creativity is a facilitator for experiencing growth after trauma (Orkibi & Ram-Vlasov, 2019), and it can help carers communicate more effectively with people with dementia in the process of co-creation (Zeilig et al., 2018). A systematic review of the impact of creativity interventions showed improvements in patient immunity, reduced visits to general practitioners, more effective pain management, and higher quality of life among people diagnosed with cancer, HIV, and other illnesses (Stuckey & Nobel, 2010). Thus, you can apply creativity throughout your life span and life conditions to enhance your health and wellbeing.

Caveat

Given that creativity is associated with risk taking, e.g. financial, health and safety, ethical, or social (Tyagi et al., 2017), make sure you keep safe when practising creativity.

References

Akinola, M., Kapadia, C., Lu, J. G., & Mason, M. F. (2019). Incorporating physiology into creativity research and practice: The effects of bodily stress responses on creativity in organizations. *Academy of Management Perspectives*, *33*(2), 163–184. https://doi-org.elib.tcd.ie/10.5465/amp.2017.0094

Beghetto, R. A., & Kaufman, J. C. (2007). The genesis of creative greatness: Mini-c and the expert performance approach. *High Ability Studies*, *18*(1), 59–61. doi:10.1080/13598130701350668.

Bolwerk, A., Mack-Andrick, J., Lang, F. R., Dörfler, A., & Maihöfner, C. (2014). How art changes your brain: Differential effects of visual art production and cognitive art evaluation on functional brain connectivity. *Public Library of Science One*, *9*(7), e101035. https://doi.org/10.1371/journal.pone.0101035

Burns, P., & Van Der Meer, R. (2021). Happy hookers: Findings from an international study exploring the effects of crochet on wellbeing. *Perspectives in Public Health*, *141*(3), 149–157. doi:10.1177/1757913920911961

Chilton, G., & Wilkinson, R. (2009). Positive art therapy: Envisioning the intersection of art therapy and positive psychology. *Australia and New Zealand Journal of Art Therapy*, *4*(1), 27–35.

Crone, D. M., O'Connell, E. E., Tyson, P. J., Clark, S. F., Opher, S., & James, D. V. B. (2013). 'Art lift' intervention to improve mental well-being: An observational study from UK general practice. *International Journal of Mental Health Nursing*, *22*(3), 279–286. https://doi-org.elib.tcd.ie/10.1111/j.1447-0349.2012.00862.x

Dalebroux, A., Goldstein, T. R., & Winner, E. (2008). Short-term mood repair through art-making: Positive emotion is more effective than venting. *Motivation & Emotion*, *32*(4), 288–295. https://doi-org.elib.tcd.ie/10.1007/s11031-008-9105-1

Forgeard, M. J. C., & Eichner, K. V. (2014). Creativity as a target and tool for positive interventions. In A. C. Parks & S. M. Schueller (Eds.), *The Wiley Blackwell handbook of positive psychological interventions* (pp. 137–154). Wiley Blackwell. https://doi.org/10.1002/9781118315927.ch7

Fredrickson, B. L., Mancuso, R. A., Branigan, C., & Tugade, M. M. (2000). The undoing effect of positive emotions. *Motivation & Emotion*, *24*(4), 237–258. https://doi-org.elib.tcd.ie/10.1023/A:1010796329158

Keller, H. (1903). *Optimism*. The Merrymount Press.

Orkibi, H., & Ram-Vlasov, N. (2019). Linking trauma to posttraumatic growth and mental health through emotional and cognitive creativity. *Psychology of Aesthetics, Creativity, and the Arts*, *13*(4), 416–430. https://doi.org/10.1037/aca0000193

Paek, S. H., Abdulla, A. M., & Cramond, B. (2016). A meta-analysis of the relationship between three common psychopathologies – ADHD, anxiety, and depression – And indicators of little-c creativity. *Gifted Child Quarterly, 60*, 117–133. doi:10.1177/0016986216630600

Saggar, M., Quintin, E.-M., Kienitz, E., Bott, N. T., Sun, Z., Hong, W.-C., Chien, Y., Liu, N., Dougherty, R. F., Royalty, A., Hawthorne, G., & Reiss, A. L. (2015). Pictionary-based fMRI paradigm to study the neural correlates of spontaneous improvisation and figural creativity. *Scientific Reports, 5*, 10894. https://doi-org.elib.tcd.ie/10.1038/srep10894

Schwenke, D., Dshemuchadse, M., Rasehorn, L., Klarhölter, D., & Scherbaum, S. (2021). Improv to improve: The impact of improvisational theater on creativity, acceptance, and psychological well-being. *Journal of Creativity in Mental Health, 16*(1), 31–48. doi:10.1080/15401383.2020.1754987

Simonton, D. K. (2021). Creativity. In C. R. Snyder, S. J. Lopez, L. M., Edwards, & S. C. Marques (Eds.), *Oxford handbook of positive psychology* (3rd ed., pp. 357–367). Oxford University Press.

Stuckey, H. L., & Nobel, J. (2010). The connection between art, healing, and public health: A review of current literature. *American Journal of Public Health, 100*(2), 254–263. https://doi.org/10.2105/AJPH.2008.156497

Tyagi, V., Hanoch, Y., Hall, S. D., Runco, M., & Denham, S. L. (2017). The risky side of creativity: Domain specific risk taking in creative individuals. *Frontiers in Psychology, 8*. https://doi-org.elib.tcd.ie/10.3389/fpsyg.2017.00145

Zeilig, H., West, J., & van der Byl Williams, M. (2018). Co-creativity: Possibilities for using the arts with people with a dementia. *Quality in Ageing & Older Adults, 19*(2), 135–145. https://doi-org.elib.tcd.ie/10.1108/QAOA-02-2018-0008

Zhao, R., Tang, Z., Lu, F., Xing, Q., & Shen, W. (2022). An updated evaluation of the dichotomous link between creativity and mental health. *Frontiers in Psychiatry, 12*, 781961. https://doi.org/10.3389/fpsyt.2021.781961

Green care

How did Miss Marple in Agatha Christie's novels solve crimes? With knitting and gardening – she claimed. Gardening has long been perceived as a hobby many have taken up for relaxation. Before research provided data, anecdotal evidence poured in from all parts of the world and suggested something special about gardening that supported healthy living. Some claimed that they drew the benefits of gardening from being outdoors; others talked about gardening as a source of physical activity; and some marvelled over the aesthetic aspects of gardening, the beauty of flowers or foliage that made them happier. Regardless of the subjective outcomes, the nexus of all gardening activities creates a special place that enhances our wellbeing and overall health. Green care refers to gardening, horticulture, and looking after plants. The difference between gardening and horticulture is that horticulture activities include looking after plants, while gardening (e.g. keeping your lawn healthy) does not necessarily include plants. Also, you can look after plants (e.g. flowers, herbs, vegetables, fruit) indoors or outdoors. Therefore, green care extends beyond a garden.

Research-based tools

Tool 20: 30 minutes of gardening (adapted from van den Berg & Custers, 2011)

When you experience a stressful event, go outdoors and garden for 30 minutes.

Tool 21: Care of plants (adapted from Kotozaki, 2014)

Buy a gardening kit, plant and take care of flowers/vegetables/herbs for at least 1 month, be it indoors or outdoors.

Tool 22: Group gardening activity (adapted from Kotozaki, 2014)

Sign up for horticultural lessons in a group setting to learn topics that might include designing a garden planter, seeding, watering, weeding, and picking flowers.

Variation of practice

There are therapeutic horticultural programmes run by trained professionals that are well researched and beneficial. Explore the programmes available in your geographic area.

Check out other tools in this book

Nature tools are associated with green care and are worth exploring. When it comes to designing your garden, combine this activity with your Creativity tools.

Mental and physical health benefits

Horticulture therapy has been shown to benefit mood (Gonzalez et al., 2010), quality of life, and general mental health, not to mention physiological health, such as reducing cortisol (stress hormone) levels (Kotozaki, 2014). In a study that put participants under stress, those who engaged in outdoor gardening soon experienced significant improvement in buoyant mood and decreased cortisol compared with participants who went indoors to read a book (van den Berg & Custers, 2011). Those who read indoors (garden view) had an increase of negative mood, which may have been due to the fact that they missed out on being outdoors. In another study, 12 weeks of therapeutic horticulture had a clinically significant decrease in depression for 50% of participants; these gains were maintained into the 3-month follow-up (Gonzalez et al., 2010). This study also highlighted participants' improvement in attention, thus demonstrating that benefits go beyond mood.

Furthermore, research indicates that horticultural activities carried out in groups are particularly beneficial, as they lead to socialisation, group solidarity, and engagement with the local community, which further impact people's wellbeing (Harris, 2017). Daily gardening is also associated with a 36% reduction in dementia symptoms (Simons et al., 2006). Gardening is particularly beneficial for the ageing population, as it allows them physical activity and leads to a range of other benefits, such as reducing pain, falls and results in lowering medication (Detweiler et al., 2012).

What often matters to our health is the presence of plants. Researchers introduced a range of potted plants in the common areas along the corridors in an experiment carried out in a residential rehabilitation centre for coronary and pulmonary patients (Raanaas et al., 2010). Residents' wellbeing was measured beforehand, 2 weeks and 4 weeks later. Patients' physical and mental health has improved following the introduction of plants and its beneficial effect was maintained one month later. In another study, when researchers compared the impact of planting seeds and planting plants (flowers), those who planted flowers (blindfolded) showed a significant reduction in blood pressure, and their brain waves indicated more profound relaxation compared to those who planted seeds (Hassan et al., 2018). Therefore, caring for plants has the potential of enhancing our wellbeing and health, not to mention making our environment so much more beautiful.

Caveat

Much research studied the effects of therapeutic horticultural programmes run by trained professionals. Such interventions span several weeks (11–20 weeks on average), lasting 60 to 120 minutes. This suggests that we would need to engage regularly and for at least 1 hour weekly to see the benefits of this type of intervention (Park et al., 2016). However, if you can't attend a programme, hopefully a short Green Care tool from this book may provide you with some positive results.

References

Detweiler, M. B., Sharma, T., Detweiler, J. G., Murphy, P. F., Lane, S., Carman, J., Chudhary, A. S., Halling, M. H., & Kim, K. Y. (2012). What is the evidence to support the use of therapeutic gardens for the elderly? *Psychiatry Investigation, 9*(2), 100–110. https://doi.org/10.4306/pi.2012.9.2.100

Gonzalez, M. T., Hartig, T., Patil, G. G., Martinsen, E. W., & Kirkevold, M. (2010). Therapeutic horticulture in clinical depression: A prospective study of active components. *Journal of Advanced Nursing, 66*(9), 2002–2013.

Harris, H. (2017). The social dimensions of therapeutic horticulture. *Health & Social Care in the Community, 25*(4), 1328–1336.

Hassan, A., Qibing, C., & Tao, J. (2018). Physiological and psychological effects of gardening activity in older adults. *Geriatrics & Gerontology International, 18*(8), 1147–1152. https://doi-org.elib.tcd.ie/10.1111/ggi.13327

Kotozaki, Y. (2014). Comparison of the effects of individual and group horticulture interventions. *Health Care: Current Reviews*, 1–5.

Park, S., Lee, A., Lee, G. J., Kim, D. S., Kim, W. S., Shoemaker, C. A., & Son, K. C. (2016). Horticultural activity interventions and outcomes: A review. *Horticultural Science & Technology, 34*(4), 513–527.

Raanaas, R. K., Patil, G. G., & Hartig, T. (2010). Effects of an indoor foliage plant intervention on patient well-being during a residential rehabilitation program. *HortScience, 45*(3), 387–392. https://doi-org.elib.tcd.ie/10.21273/HORTSCI.45.3.387

Simons, L. A., Simons, J., McCallum, J., & Friedlander, Y. (2006). Lifestyle factors and risk of dementia: Dubbo study of the elderly. *The Medical Journal of Australia, 184*(2), 68–70. https://doi.org/10.5694/j.1326-5377.2006.tb00120.x

Van Den Berg, A. E., & Custers, M. H. (2011). Gardening promotes neuroendocrine and affective restoration from stress. *Journal of Health Psychology, 16*(1), 3–11. https://doi.org/10.1177/1359105310365577

Your reflection space

Which calming tools would you like to try? Why?
Which activities did you find most useful? How did you tweak them?

3 Energising tools

Energising tools are activities that require expending energy, which can paradoxically provide us with bundles of new energy. Business writers Tony Schwarz and Catherine McCarthy (2007) claimed that to get more done in the day, we do not need good time management, hiring a helper, or using a new app. Instead, we need to focus on creating more energy in our body and mind to help us attend to life more effectively.

Imagine Arjun and Sarah, two parents in full-time jobs, perpetually exhausted juggling their childcare and work. They may create a solid tag-team-parenting-type schedule that will help them manage the symptoms of their exhaustion, but unless they get to the bottom of it and work on expanding their energies at the source, they will continue to be stuck in a vicious cycle. To get unstuck and change their vicious cycle into a healthy cycle, they can go back to the basics and develop ways to keep their bodies healthy and energised so that they have the strength to juggle. This may include waking up half an hour earlier to exercise, changing their sleep pattern, or ensuring they get the nutrition that sustains their high energy expenditure.

The body seems to work on a simple basis of "use it or lose it". Therefore, if we exercise by engaging in movement of almost any kind, the body will assume that this will continue well into the future and help support us in the process. The result will be balanced energy storage, less accumulation of fat, stronger muscles, more flexible limbs, efficient food digestion, and expanded lung and heart capacities. All these processes make us feel better and more energetic. Energising tools like exercise can also help us stay in the present moment, which can be an effective antidote to anxiety, low mood, and overthinking that often deplete our energy resources.

This chapter provides various tools to help you find more energy in life.

DOI: 10.4324/9781003279594-5

Energising tools include:

1. Physical activity
2. Blue spaces
3. Nutrition
4. Play
5. Humour

Reference

Schwarz, T., & McCarthy, C. (2007). Manage your energy, not your time. *Harvard Business Review*. https://hbr.org/2007/10/manage-your-energy-not-your-time

Physical activity

Physical activity (moderate intensity) refers to any bodily movement that gets our hearts pumping and results in energy expenditure and breaking a sweat (Acevedo, 2012). This includes the whole range of daily activities, such as climbing the stairs, making dinner, walking the dog, cleaning, shopping, playing with children, etc. On the other hand, exercise (vigorous-intensity aerobic activity) is a more structured activity that aims to maintain or improve physical fitness or health (Acevedo, 2012). According to the World Health Organisation (WHO, 2018), one in four adults and three in four adolescents do not meet the global recommendations for physical activity. Adults (18–65 years) are required to have weekly 150 to 300 minutes of moderate-intensity, or 75 to 150 minutes of vigorous-intensity aerobic activity, or a combination of both; older adults (65+ years) are recommended to do three or more days of moderate or greater intensity, multicomponent (functional balance and strength training) physical activity; children and adolescents (5–17 years) are required to do 60 minutes of moderate to vigorous aerobic activity (Bull et al., 2020). The 19th-century Prussian philosopher Wilhelm Von Humboldt wrote that mind and body are always united, and the true enjoyment in life comes from exercising both body and mind.

Research-based tools

Tool 23: Relish your household chores (adapted from Crum & Langer, 2007)

We can break household chores into low and high intensity. Low intensity includes:

Washing the dishes, dusting
Making the bed

Doing the laundry
Hanging out the laundry, ironing
Tidying up and cooking meals

High intensity includes activities such as:

Window cleaning
Changing the bed
Vacuuming, washing the floor, and
Home-improvement jobs like general home DIY.

Household chores can help us keep fit and lose weight. How might you conduct a different approach to your household chores? It is all about perspective and mindset. For example, if you approach vacuum cleaning as a painful, meaningless experience that you wish someone else would do, it will become so. On the other hand, if you approach the same task as a means to extend your longevity and stave off illness, as well as a reason not to go to the gym, then you might have a very different experience.

This experiment was conducted with hotel cleaning staff and showed that mindset, not the activity, positively affected participants' health.

Tool 24: Daily activity records (adapted from Speck & Looney, 2001)

All you are asked to do is complete daily activity records for 12 weeks. First, you note any activity you engaged in for the day, be it walking, chores, childcare, or others. You also need to note the intensity of your activity, i.e. if it was moderate or vigorous. Finally, you are asked to use a pedometer, and when completing your daily activity records, you are asked to note how many steps you have taken during the day. This simple activity resulted in participants' significant increase in physical activity.

Tool 25: Aerobic and yoga exercise (used with permission from Herbert et al., 2020)

Twice a week over the next 6 weeks, block out 8 to 16 minutes (depending on your fitness level) and conduct one of the following options for an aerobic exercise:

Option 1

Warm-up: run on the spot (20 sec), turn in hips while running (15 sec), stand upright, hands on hips, and do a butt-kick exercise (15 sec), windmill arm rotation exercise (20 sec)

Exercise (30/45/60 sec per exercise for intensity 1, 2, or 3): raise arms overhead, air punches to the side, air punches to the front, front kicks, high knees, diagonal kicks, wrist/toe touches

Cooldown: run on the spot, shake out arms (15 sec), standing straddle stretch with arms hanging loose (15 sec), upper-body twist and dynamic stretching to the side (15 sec), upper-body twist, stretching to the side including arms (15 sec)

Option 2

Warm-up: hop on the spot (20 sec), turn in hips while jumping (15 sec), stand upright, hands on hips, and do a butt-kick exercise (15 sec), arms to the front while jumping (20 sec)

Exercise (30/45/60 sec per exercise for intensity 1, 2, or 3): arm circles, uppercuts, overhead (air) punches, lateral jumps/side-to-side jumps with arms crossed, squat with side taps, x jumps, arm circles

Cooldown: wiggle on tiptoe, lift heels (15 sec), standing straddle stretch, shake out thighs (15 sec), arms reach slowly overhead, stretching arms (15 sec), upper-body twist, stretching to the side including arms (15 sec)

Please make sure you alternate arms, legs, and sides as you carry out your exercise. Also, please note that this series of aerobic exercises was tested with younger people, i.e. university students. Don't hesitate to contact your general practitioner for advice on age- and fitness-appropriate aerobic exercise before you replicate it.

Tool 26: Community-based exercise (adapted from Burke et al., 2006)

Exercising in a safe group versus exercising alone can help us better achieve our goals related to physical movement. Exercising in a safe group of like-minded individuals makes us feel part of a tribe with a common goal. In addition, group activities activate our social engagement system, which positively affects stress management. The list of group-based exercises is almost endless and includes team-based sports, class-based programmes, and local clubs.

Variations of practice

Apart from the activities mentioned, you can select a range of other aerobic exercises, e.g. swimming, cycling, walking, rowing) and engage with them regularly. The ever-expanding number of commercially available smart devices out there can help some of us achieve our goals related to movement and exercise. Smartphone apps, phones, wearable devices, and watches are available in the marketplace, many of which offer myriad ways to track and measure your movement and exercise. Many find it helpful that their household chores and activities like simply walking to the shops can be added to daily exercise requirements. It can be nice to see that activity you never regarded as exercise or "gym work" can be recorded and added to your daily movement needs for health. However, for some, these devices can lead to obsessive checking and anxiety, while others still find their incessant reminders an annoyance and a hindrance to daily exercise. As ever, it is up to you to decide what is best for you.

Try conscious exercise practices like yoga rather than running on a treadmill while watching the news. What do we mean by conscious exercise? Exercise that involves paying attention to the body in the present moment. We can engage in conscious exercise of any kind when we pay attention using a mindful approach. For example, we run consciously when we pay attention to our heart beating, feet hitting the ground, and our skin temperature. We can also engage in more established conscious exercise programmes through yoga (Wieland et al., 2021), tai chi, and many martial arts (Bu et al., 2010).

Recent psychological research shows that the perception of difficulty associated with exercise depends on the individual's attention (Balcetis et al., 2020). If you find exercising difficult, try this activity when exercising: Usually, when you exercise, your attention is drawn towards the world around you. For example, when you are walking or running, you pass by people or places which may distract you. When this happens, you will find the exercise more challenging to do. Instead, focus your attention on something ahead of you allow and all other people and objects to dissolve. Once you reach the place you are focused on, select another focus point ahead of you, letting all other things around it dissolve. Continue exercising like this, as it will make your exercise easier to do.

Emerging research suggests that Marie Kondo's decluttering method may also increase wellbeing concerning household chores used as physical activity (Hsin-Hsuan, 2017). It is associated with a highly structured approach to regular decluttering and tidying the house. However, limited research is available about its effect on psychological or physical wellbeing.

Check out other tools in this book

Blue Spaces tools provide additional ideas on how to carry out physical activity. Also, Nutrition tools are complementary to physical activity.

Mental and physical health benefits

It is accepted that exercise is essential for longevity (Kopp & Burtscher, 2021) and good health (Ruegsegger & Booth, 2018). Less understood is the importance of exercise for our mental health and general wellbeing. Mounting research has shown that exercise strongly affects our physiology, improving our cardiometabolic health and reducing mortality (Chastin et al., 2019). It also affects our biology, sense of purpose, cognitive functioning, and emotional regulation (Mandolesi et al., 2018). A study with more than 14,000 American adults showed that physical activity was associated with a greater sense of purpose in life when examined over 4 years (Yemiscigil & Vlaev, 2021). This was especially true for older adults. Likewise, moderate aerobic exercise positively impacts emotional regulation, self-esteem, positive body image, self-control, sexual satisfaction, and general wellbeing (Mandolesi et al., 2018). Engaging in a high-intensity exercise as presented in tool 25 over a month and a half was associated with a decline in symptoms of depression, overall perceived stress, and stress due to uncertainty, as well as improvement of wellbeing, not to mention cardiovascular health (Herbert et al., 2020).

Regular physical activity is associated with academic performance (Singh et al., 2019). In addition, strong evidence suggests it reduces anxiety and depression and enhances students' self-esteem (Dale et al., 2018). Among adults, physical activity, e.g. walking or running, is also one of the most effective preventative measures against depression (Mammen & Faulkner, 2013) and a treatment for it (Bailey et al., 2018). Furthermore, it prevents cognitive decline in Alzheimer-type dementia (Brasure et al., 2018). It helps patients reduce their symptoms of illness or enhance the quality of life in such conditions as multiple sclerosis (Kalb et al., 2020), cardiovascular disease (Prabhu et al., 2020), diabetes (Zaharieva et al., 2020), and rheumatoid arthritis (Khoja et al., 2018), to mention but a few.

Exercise is not the only way to increase physical activity. Lessons from the Blue Zone Initiative, where humans live the longest (Buettner & Skemp, 2016), and recent research (Lee et al., 2021) show that engaging in household chores can also contribute to longevity and health. Household chores are associated with a range of benefits that go beyond keeping your home clean and tidy. When older people engage in household chores, they report higher wellbeing, better physical health, and sleep quality (Rodriguez-Stanley et al., 2020). Furthermore, keeping your home tidy keeps your legs strong, which prevents trips and falls, not to mention increased cognitive health (Lee et al., 2021). Finally, your mindset matters when it comes to doing your household chores.

In an experiment with cleaning staff across seven hotels, the researchers found that those who firmly believed that their job of cleaning could help them keep fit and healthy saw a decrease in weight, blood pressure, body fat, waist-to-hip ratio, and body mass index (Crum & Langer, 2007). Thus, changing your attitude towards your daily chores can improve your health.

Furthermore, simple activities that encourage us to self-monitor our physical activity, such as the previously mentioned daily record of activities (e.g. Speck & Looney, 2001), are among the most effective ways to increase physical activity (Michie et al., 2009). You can mix and match it with any physical activity to achieve your goals.

Caveats

Please note that before you engage in exercise or a more intense form of physical activity, visit your general practitioner or healthcare provider, especially if you have not exercised for a while. Get expert advice, and take things slowly. Three conditions, in particular, require medical attention while practising exercise, i.e. myocardial infarction (heart attack), musculoskeletal injury, and exercise dependence, which is a psychological condition characterised by a strong perceived need to engage in exercise (Hefferon, 2013). However, these three conditions are not exhaustive, so visit your doctor before engaging in an exercise of any kind. You may have heard about the 10,000-steps-a-day recommendation. However, the original study in Japan recommended a range of steps depending on the individual's circumstances; an average child might do as many as 15,000 a day, whilst an average older adult or a person with an illness might do significantly fewer. Therefore, make sure you build up your steps systematically rather than overstraining yourself if you use any pedometer programmes. When selecting a community group, think about safety first and ensure the group you are joining is trustworthy.

References

Acevedo, E. (2012). Exercise psychology: Understanding the mental health benefits of physical activity and the public health challenges of inactivity. In E. Acevado (Ed.), *The Oxford Handbook of Exercise Psychology* (pp. 3–8). Oxford University Press.

Bailey, A., Hetrick, S., Rosenbaum, S., Purcell, R., & Parker, A. (2018). Treating depression with physical activity in adolescents and young adults: A systematic review and meta-analysis of randomised controlled trials. *Psychological Medicine*, *48*(7), 1068–1083. doi:10.1017/S0033291717002653

Balcetis, E., Riccio, M. T., Duncan, D. T., & Cole, S. (2020). Keeping the goal in sight: Testing the influence of narrowed visual attention on physical activity. *Personality & Social Psychology Bulletin*, *46*(3), 485–496. https://doi-org.elib.tcd.ie/10.1177/0146167219861438

Brasure, M., Desai, P., Davila, H., Nelson, V. A., Calvert, C., Jutkowitz, E., Butler, M., Fink, H. A., Ratner, E., Hemmy, L. S., McCarten, J. R., Barclay, T. R., & Kane, R. L. (2018). Physical activity interventions in preventing cognitive decline and Alzheimer-type dementia: A systematic review. *Annals of Internal Medicine*, *168*(1), 30–38. https://doi-org.elib.tcd.ie/10.7326/M17-1528

Bu, B., Haijun, H., Yong, L., Chaohui, Z., Xiaoyuan, Y., & Singh, M. F. (2010). Effects of martial arts on health status: A systematic review. *Journal of Evidence-Based Medicine*, *3*(4), 205–219. doi:10.1111/j.1756-5391.2010.01107.x

Buettner, D., & Skemp, S. (2016). Blue zones: Lessons from the world's longest lived. *American Journal of Lifestyle Medicine*, *10*(5), 318–321. doi:10.1177/1559827616637066

Bull, F. C., Al-Ansari, S. S., Biddle, S., Borodulin, K., Buman, M. P., Cardon, G., Carty, C., Chaput, J. P., Chastin, S., Chou, R., Dempsey, P. C., DiPietro, L., Ekelund, U., Firth, J., Friedenreich, C. M., Garcia, L., Gichu, M., Jago, R., Katzmarzyk, P. T., Lambert, E., . . . Willumsen, J. F. (2020). World health organization 2020 guidelines on physical activity and sedentary behaviour. *British Journal of Sports Medicine*, *54*(24), 1451–1462. https://doi.org/10.1136/bjsports-2020-102955

Burke, S. M., Carrón, A. V., Eys, M. A., Ntoumanis, N., & Estabrooks, P. A. (2006). Group versus individual approach? A meta-analysis of the effectiveness of interventions to promote physical activity. *International Review of Sport and Exercise Psychology*, *2*(1), 13.

Chastin, S. F. M., De Craemer, M., De Cocker, K., Powell, L., Van Cauwenberg, J., Dall, P., Hamer, M., & Stamatakis, E. (2019). How does light-intensity physical activity associate with adult cardiometabolic health and mortality? Systematic review with meta-analysis of experimental and observational studies. *British Journal of Sports Medicine*, *53*(6), 370–376. https://doi-org.elib.tcd.ie/10.1136/bjsports-2017-097563

Crum, A. J., & Langer, E. J. (2007). Mind-set matters: Exercise and the placebo effect. *Psychological Science*, *18*(2), 165–171. https://doi.org/10.1111/j.1467-9280.2007.01867.x

Dale, L. P., Vanderloo, L., Moore, S., & Faulkner, G. (2019). Physical activity and depression, anxiety, and self-esteem in children and youth: An umbrella systematic review. *Mental Health and Physical Activity*, *16*, 66–79. https://doi-org.elib.tcd.ie/10.1016/j.mhpa.2018.12.001

Hefferon, K. (2013). *Positive psychology and the body: The somatopsychic side to flourishing*. The Open University Press.

Hsin-Hsuan Meg Lee. (2017). In pursuit of happiness: Phenomenological study of the Konmari decluttering method. *Advances in Consumer Research*, *45*, 454–457.

Kalb, R., Brown, T. R., Coote, S., Costello, K., Dalgas, U., Garmon, E., Giesser, B., Halper, J., Karpatkin, H., Keller, J., Ng, A. V., Pilutti, L. A., Rohrig, A., Van Asch, P., Zackowski, K., & Motl, R. W. (2020). Exercise and lifestyle physical activity recommendations for people with multiple sclerosis throughout the disease course. *Multiple Sclerosis Journal, 26*(12), 1459–1469. https://doi-org.elib.tcd.ie/10.1177/1352458520915629

Khoja, S. S., Moore, C. G., Goodpaster, B. H., Delitto, A., & Piva, S. R. (2018). Skeletal muscle fat and its association with physical function in rheumatoid arthritis. *Arthritis Care & Research, 70*(3), 333–342. https://doi-org.elib.tcd.ie/10.1002/acr.23278

Kopp, M., & Burtscher, M. (2021). Aiming at optimal physical activity for longevity (OPAL). *Sports Medicine – Open, 7*(1), 70. doi:10.1186/s40798-021-00360-4

Lee, S. Y., Pang, B. W. J., Lau, L. K., Jabbar, K. A., Seah, W. T., Chen, K. K., . . . Wee, S.-L. (2021). Cross-sectional associations of housework with cognitive, physical and sensorimotor functions in younger and older community-dwelling adults: The Yishun Study. *BMJ Open, 11*(11), e052557. doi:10.1136/bmjopen-2021-052557

Mammen, G., & Faulkner, G. (2013). Physical activity and the prevention of depression: A systematic review of prospective studies. *American Journal of Preventive Medicine, 45*(5), 649–657. https://doi-org.elib.tcd.ie/10.1016/j.amepre.2013.08.001

Mandolesi, L., Polverino, A., Montuori, S., Foti, F., Ferraioli, G., Sorrentino, P., & Sorrentino, G. (2018). Effects of physical exercise on cognitive functioning and wellbeing: Biological and psychological benefits. *Frontiers in Psychology, 9*(509). doi:10.3389/fpsyg.2018.00509

Michie, S., Abraham, C., Whittington, C., McAteer, J., & Gupta, S. (2009). Effective techniques in healthy eating and physical activity interventions: A meta-regression. *Health Psychology, 28*(6), 690–701. https://doi.org/10.1037/a0016136

Prabhu, N. V., Maiya, A. G., & Prabhu, N. S. (2020). Impact of cardiac rehabilitation on functional capacity and physical activity after coronary revascularization: A scientific review. *Cardiology Research & Practice*, 1–9. https://doi-org.elib.tcd.ie/10.1155/2020/1236968

Rodriguez-Stanley, J., Alonso-Ferres, M., Zilioli, S., & Slatcher, R. B. (2020). Housework, health, and wellbeing in older adults: The role of socioeconomic status. *Journal of Family Psychology: JFP: Journal of the Division of Family Psychology of the American Psychological Association* (Division 43), *34*(5), 610–620. https://doi.org/10.1037/fam0000630

Ruegsegger, G. N., & Booth, F. W. (2018). Health benefits of exercise. *Cold Spring Harbor Perspectives in Medicine, 8*(7), a029694. doi:10.1101/cshperspect.a029694

Singh, A. S., Saliasi, E., van den Berg, V., Uijtdewilligen, L., de Groot, R. H. M., Jolles, J., Andersen, L. B., Bailey, R., Chang, Y.-K., Diamond, A., Ericsson, I., Etnier, J. L., Fedewa, A. L., Hillman, C. H., McMorris, T., Pesce, C., Pühse, U., Tomporowski, P. D., & Chinapaw, M. J. M. (2019). Effects of physical activity interventions on cognitive and academic performance in children and adolescents: A novel combination of a systematic review and recommendations from an expert panel. *British Journal of Sports Medicine, 53*(10), 640–647. https://doi-org.elib.tcd.ie/10.1136/bjsports-2017-098136

Speck, B. J., & Looney, S. W. (2001). Effects of a minimal intervention to increase physical activity in women: Daily activity records. *Nursing Research, 50*(6), 374–378. https://doi.org/10.1097/00006199-200111000-00008

WHO. (2018). *Global action plan on physical activity 2018–2030: More active people for a healthier world*. WHO.

Wieland, L. S., Cramer, H., Lauche, R., Verstappen, A., Parker, E. A., & Pilkington, K. (2021). Evidence on yoga for health: A bibliometric analysis of systematic reviews. *Complementary Therapies in Medicine*, *60*, 102746. https://doi.org/10.1016/j.ctim.2021.102746

Yemiscigil, A., & Vlaev, I. (2021). The bidirectional relationship between sense of purpose in life and physical activity: A longitudinal study. *Journal of Behavioral Medicine*, *44*(5), 715–725. doi:10.1007/s10865-021-00220-2

Zaharieva, D. P., McGaugh, S., Davis, E. A., & Riddell, M. C. (2020). Advances in exercise, physical activity, and diabetes. *Diabetes Technology & Therapeutics*, *22*, S-109–S-118. https://doi-org.elib.tcd.ie/10.1089/dia.2020.2508

Blue spaces

The Sea, the Sea (written by Iris Murdoch) and *The Old Man and the Sea* (written by Ernest Hemingway) are two of many depictions of the literary authors' love for blue spaces. Literary fiction and folk tales have long appreciated the beauty of the sea and its calming effect. However, only recently have psychologists begun to explore the benefits of water spaces for physical health and wellbeing. Research on blue spaces extends beyond the impact of nature in general. Blue spaces refer to visible outdoor water environments, such as the sea, lakes, rivers, streams; they exclude outdoor swimming pools, garden ponds, or fountains (Britton et al., 2020). Spending time in blue spaces provides some of the up-and-coming tools that can enhance the wellbeing of nations given free access to water resources.

Research-based tools

Tool 27: Get active (Britton et al., 2020)

Engage in one of the following activities in blue spaces:

- Beach activity
- Canoeing
- Dragon boat racing
- Fly-fishing
- Kayaking
- Sailing
- Scuba diving
- Surfing
- Swimming

These tools can be used as a single-day activity or ongoing.

Variations of practice

Consider any other water sports that are not mentioned. Also, whilst there is very little research about the impact of walking, running, or swimming in the context of blue spaces (Foley & Kistemann, 2015), there is plenty of evidence to suggest that these activities, regardless of whether they are conducted in blue spaces, can boost wellbeing and health. Therefore, they are also recommended. Furthermore, research has recently emerged about the positive impact of simple skygazing (Conway & Hefferon, 2019). Given that people often engage voluntarily in seagazing, it may have a similar effect on wellbeing as skygazing. Hopefully, future research will explore it further and identify blue-space gazing as one of the interventions for wellbeing. Another option is cold-water immersion (cold water, ice or winter swimming). During winter, it refers to swimming outdoors in colder and even polar regions, in water below 50 °C, and some cases below 100 °C (Knechtle et al., 2020). Immersion comes with a range of benefits (see what follows); however, it may be risky (e.g. Tipton et al., 2017); thus take care to acclimatise adequately. Please consult your doctor and cold-water immersion clubs and societies in your area, as well as evidence-based resources, such as a guide on how to acclimatise to cold water (Massey & Scully, 2022), before attempting to do it. There are plenty of studies showing the benefits of it. However, we are still waiting for an experiment to identify the clear-cut impact of cold-water immersion on various aspects of wellbeing.

Check out other tools in this book

Review Nature and Horticulture tools for additional ideas.

Mental and physical health benefits

The most significant benefit noted across more than 30 studies using Blue Space tools was the positive impact that blue spaces had on mental health and psychosocial wellbeing (Britton et al., 2020). This included an enhanced sense of connection with others, self-esteem, self-efficacy, and resilience. Furthermore, engaging in water activities was associated with a more positive body image (McDonough et al., 2008) and enhanced self-concept (Capurso & Borsci, 2013). Individuals living near the sea report higher health and wellbeing levels than those living away from the sea (White et al., 2016). Furthermore, cold-water swimming demonstrates various psychological benefits, such as refocusing the mind on the *here and now* and coping with anxiety and depression (Oliver, 2021). Being in the vicinity of water is not only aesthetically appealing but can be good for your mental health.

From the physiological perspective, water sport participation was associated with a significant drop in heart rate and improved participant fitness (Hignett et al., 2017). The benefits of blue spaces have been recognised for people with disability. For example, a surf programme for young people with disability showed improvement in their physical as well as psychosocial wellbeing (Britton et al., 2020), while amputees and participants with burn and brain injuries reported that surfing helped them manage their pain and improve their mobility (Fleischmann et al., 2011). Cold-water immersion, in particular, is associated with a range of physiological benefits such as insulin metabolism, helping individuals lose weight (Gibas-Dorna et al., 2016), and improved immunity (Brazaitis et al., 2014).

Caveats

As with all sports, please consult a medical professional before engaging with physical activity. Also, practice safety when in water. When possible, engage with all water activities in the company of others. Finally, adverse effects were noted in some studies, which included seasickness (Britton et al., 2020), fatigue in cancer survivors (e.g. McDonough et al., 2008), and lower mood in participants with PTSD (Caddick et al., 2015). Therefore, please use these tools with caution. Finally, cold-water immersion may act as a precursor to drowning, cardiac arrest, or hypothermia (Tipton et al., 2017) and thus should be used with caution.

References

Brazaitis, M., Eimantas, N., Daniuseviciute, L., Mickeviciene, D., Steponaviciute, R., & Skurvydas, A. (2014). Two strategies for response to 14 °C cold-water immersion: Is there a difference in the response of motor, cognitive, immune and stress markers? *PLoS One, 9*.

Britton, E., Kindermann, G., Domegan, C., & Carlin, C. (2020). Blue care: A systematic review of blue space interventions for health and wellbeing. *Health Promotion International, 35*(1), 50–69. https://doi-org.elib.tcd.ie/10.1093/heapro/day103

Caddick, N., Smith, B., & Phoenix, C. (2015). The effects of surfing and the natural environment on the wellbeing of combat veterans. *Qualitative Health Research, 25*, 76–86.

Capurso, M., & Borsci, S. (2013). Effects of a tall ship sail training experience on adolescents' self-concept. *International Journal of Educational Research, 58*, 15–24.

Conway, P., & Hefferon, K. (2019). *The extraordinary in the ordinary: Skychology – An interpretative phenomenological analysis of looking up at the sky.* Retrieved from: https://www.researchgate.net/profile/Paul-Conway-3/publication/331702864_The_extraordinary_in_the_ordinary_Skychology_-_an_interpretative_phenomenological_analysis_of_looking_up_at_the_sky/links/5ea1491ba6fdcc88fc362c82/The-extraordinary-in-the-ordinary-Skychology-an-interpretative-phenomenological-analysis-of-looking-up-at-the-sky.pdf

Fleischmann, D., Michalewicz, B., Stedje-Larsen, E., Neff, J., Murphy, J., Browning, K., et al. (2011). Surf medicine: Surfing as a means of therapy for combat-related polytrauma. *Journal of Prosthetics and Orthotics, 23*, 27–29.

Foley, R., & Kistemann, T. (2015). Blue space geographies: Enabling health in place. *Health & Place, 35*, 157–165. https://doi.org/10.1016/j.healthplace.2015.07.003

Gibas-Dorna, M., Checińska, Z., Korek, E., Kupsz, J., Sowińska, A., & Krauss, H. (2016). Cold water swimming beneficially modulates insulin sensitivity in middle-aged individuals. *Journal of Aging & Physical Activity, 24*(4), 547–554. https://doi-org.elib.tcd.ie/10.1123/japa.2015-0222

Hignett, A., White, M. P., Pahl, S., Jenkin, R., & Froy, M. L. (2017). Evaluation of a surfing programme designed to increase personal wellbeing and connectedness to the natural environment among at risk young people. *Journal of Adventure Education and Outdoor Learning, 18*, 53–69.

Knechtle, B., Waśkiewicz, Z., Sousa, C. V., Hill, L., & Nikolaidis, P. T. (2020). Cold water swimming – Benefits and risks: A narrative review. *International Journal of Environmental Research and Public Health, 17*(23), 8984. https://doi.org/10.3390/ijerph17238984

Massey, H., & Scully, P. (2022). *How to acclimatise to cold water: Dipping into Autumn? Here's what happens to the body of a regular swimmer.* www.outdoorswimmingsociety.com/how-to-acclimatise-to-cold-water/

McDonough, M. H., Sabiston, C. M., & Crocker, P. R. (2008). An interpretative phenomenological examination of psychosocial changes among breast cancer survivors in their first season of dragon boating. *Journal of Applied Sport Psychology, 20*, 425–440.

Oliver, B. (2021). Cold water swimming for wellbeing. *Journal of Public Mental Health, 20*(2), 105–110. https://doi-org.elib.tcd.ie/10.1108/JPMH-02-2021-0027

Tipton, M. J., Collier, N., Massey, H., Corbett, J., & Harper, M. (2017). Cold water immersion: Kill or cure. *Experimental Physiology, 102*(11), 1335–1355. doi:10.1113/EP086283

White, M. P., Pahl, S., Wheeler, B. W., Fleming, L. E. F., & Depledge, M. H. (2016). The blue gym': What can blue space do for you and what can you do for blue space? *Journal of the Marine Biological Association of the United Kingdom, 96*(1), 5–12. doi:10.1017/S0025315415002209.

Nutrition

We need food to survive. It is the fuel that keeps us going. If the fuel we consume is processed and of low quality, it will sustain our existence but will not provide us with adequate nourishment to flourish. It is just like fuel in our cars. Lousy-quality fuel will either destroy the engine or make the car sluggish. Similarly, a lousy diet will result in low energy and low mood that will prevent us from living our lives fully, not to mention that it can make our bodies sick. When we use terms like "diet" and "nutrition", we mean consuming food containing protein, complex sugars, fats, minerals, vitamins, and trace elements required for energy, repair, and maintenance of a healthy body. The right mixture of these components will keep our bodies and minds at the height of their performance.

Research-based tools

Tool 28: Blue zone diet (Buettner & Skemp, 2016)

The eating habits of blue zone inhabitants:

- Consume fewer daily calories.
- Less than 5% of the diet is comprised of meat and fish.
- Eat fresh fruit and vegetables.
- Consume beans and nuts daily.

Tool 29: Feed your brain and gut

You do not have to go out and stock up on pre- and probiotic supplements to feed the beneficial bacteria in your gut (Harvard Health, 2021). Instead, the best approach is to eat a standard healthy diet.

Eat:

- High-fibre food rich in prebiotics (food that feeds good gut bacteria) such as lentils, asparagus, beans, onions, garlic, bananas, beets, and broccoli (among others)
- Fermented food[1] – sauerkraut, kimchi, pickled vegetables and fish, fermented soy products
- Yoghurt with live bacteria

Avoid or limit consumption:

- Alcohol
- Junk food
- Processed meats
- Commercial emulsifiers (e.g. polysorbate and carboxymethylcellulose) found in ice cream

Tool 30: Cook and eat mindfully (Dunn et al., 2018).

Pay attention to the food you eat. Take time before each meal to cultivate gratitude for those who grew, cultivated, harvested, processed, delivered, and cooked this food. Be grateful for the fact that you have food to eat. Savour the texture, smell, taste, and temperature of each bite. This approach will slow down the time it takes to eat a meal and assist digestion. It might also contribute to managing healthy body weight. In a 2016 RCT (randomised controlled trial) by Daubenmier and colleagues, 194 adults were randomised into an exercise/education-based weight loss programme or the same programme plus mindful eating practice and education (Daubenmier et al., 2016). Those trained in mindful eating lost significantly more weight. The practice involves taking space and time before eating each meal, savouring each bite, including smell, texture, and taste.

Tool 31: Eat with others (Yiengprugsawan et al., 2015)

If you can, eat with others; it might make you happier. Commensalism (eating together) is common in many cultures but has declined over the past 100 years. We are all time poor, but if we can, we should carve out some space, if not daily, then at least at the weekend, to sit with other human beings and share in the joy that eating can bring. It doesn't have to be a four-course festive meal. Eat an apple with your friend. Share noodles with your kids. The critical point is to be and eat together and do it as often as possible.

Tool 32: Fruit a day (Zhong et al., 2021)

This activity benefits those who do not eat five fruits and/or vegetables daily – an excellent way to start a helpful habit. For the next 3 weeks, add a banana, an apple, or another fruit or portion of fruit to your lunch each day.

Variations of practice

If your diet is not as good as you would like it to be, add or replace one product a week. For example, if you eat chips every day, try roasting or steaming potatoes one day a week. Or if you don't eat fruit and vegetables, introduce one fruit or veg a week, then increase your intake to twice a week, every other day, and then every day.

Check out other tools in this book

Mindfulness tools can provide additional support in developing mindful eating. Also, please check Compassionate tools for guidance on how to prevent binge eating.

Mental and physical health benefits

A healthy diet promotes physical health, such as balanced immune and cardiovascular functioning. However, it also strengthens characteristics of positive psychology (Holder, 2019) that include:

- Life satisfaction
- Optimism
- Positive emotions
- Flourishing
- Motivation

Evidence from the earth's blue zones, where people live the longest, shows that diet and nutrition are essential in longevity, health, and happiness (Buettner & Skemp, 2016). The emerging evidence is clear; eating a healthy diet cultivates and sustains individual wellbeing. In a recent extensive review of existing research, Mark D. Holder from British Columbia describes strong links between what we eat and positive mental health. For example, when a group of bus drivers added a fruit a day to complement their lunch, their depressive symptoms reduced significantly, and they improved their belief in ability and road safety (Zhong et al., 2021).

Until recently, we understood little about the effect of diet on mood. Researchers are now uncovering the importance of gut bacteria (microbiome) and how they interact with the food we consume to form factors important for normal brain and nerve functioning and mood (Clapp et al., 2017). A functioning nervous system and brain require the production of chemical messengers called neurotransmitters that allow rapid transmission of messages throughout the body. For example, a humble piece of cheese contains the amino acid (building blocks of proteins) tryptophan. When we eat cheese, the beneficial bacteria in our gut, such as *Lactobacillus* and *Bifidobacterium*, can convert tryptophan into the neurotransmitter serotonin (Gao et al., 2020). Serotonin (also called a hormone) is one of the neurotransmitters responsible for positive mood in the brain. Taken together, these hormones and transmitters can communicate dissatisfaction to our brains and serve to alter our mood and subjective wellbeing. Suppose we continue to experience a poor diet, leading to a disrupted gut microbiome. In that case, we will have a persistent disruption in these neurotransmitters and hormones, which will have a subsequent negative impact on our long-term mood and sense of wellbeing. Finally, we know that eating alone is bad for your health (Björnwall et al., 2021). It might be that when we live alone, our interest in the quality and quantity of food intake decreases, thereby impacting our health as a result of poor nutritional intake. Interestingly, individuals with special dietary requirements such as type 2 diabetes and other food-related ailments often eat alone rather than with their families (Yiengprugsawan et al., 2015); this will have an added knock-on effect on their health. Furthermore, eating alone is a risk factor for developing malnutrition and lower socioeconomic status. It is also interesting to note that eating together has the most significant positive impact on older adults (Yiengprugsawan et al., 2015).

Caveats

Information surrounding diet and nutrition can change dramatically, often with conflicting messages. This is especially the case for emerging diet programmes for weight loss. It is best to follow the example of those who live the longest (those who live in blue zones) by eating less meat and processed food while eating more fresh fruit, vegetables, nuts, and beans. The Blue Zone Initiative promotes a Mediterranean diet for health and longevity. However, it is not always possible or feasible for many to eat such a diet. For example, growing tomatoes and olives is slim in Ireland! Look out for healthy equivalents where you live. In Ireland, we have access to fresh root vegetables, nuts, berries, good seafood, and superfoods such as seaweed. Create your region-specific version of the Mediterranean diet, and you will not go wrong. Finally, be careful when consuming fermented food if you have irritable bowel syndrome or are immunocompromised. Check with your healthcare provider before eating.

Note

1 Some commercially available fermented food products like sauerkraut are pasteurised, which kills beneficial bacteria.

References

Björnwall, A., Mattsson Sydner, Y., Koochek, A., & Neuman, N. (2021). Eating alone or together among community-living older people-a scoping review. *International*

Journal of Environmental Research and Public Health, 18(7), 3495. doi:10.3390/ijerph18073495

Buettner, D., & Skemp, S. (2016). Blue zones: Lessons from the world's longest lived. *American Journal of Lifestyle Medicine*, 10(5), 318–321. doi:10.1177/1559827616637066

Clapp, M., Aurora, N., Herrera, L., Bhatia, M., Wilen, E., & Wakefield, S. (2017). Gut microbiota's effect on mental health: The gut-brain axis. *Clinics and Practice*, 7(4), 987–987. doi:10.4081/cp.2017.987

Daubenmier, J., Moran, P. J., Kristeller, J., Acree, M., Bacchetti, P., Kemeny, M. E., ... Hecht, F. M. (2016). Effects of a mindfulness-based weight loss intervention in adults with obesity: A randomized clinical trial. *Obesity*, 24(4), 794–804. https://doi.org/10.1002/oby.21396

Dunn, C., Haubenreiser, M., Johnson, M., Nordby, K., Aggarwal, S., Myer, S., & Thomas, C. (2018). Mindfulness approaches and weight loss, weight maintenance, and weight regain. *Current Obesity Reports*, 7(1), 37–49. doi:10.1007/s13679-018-0299-6

Gao, K., Mu, C.-L., Farzi, A., & Zhu, W.-Y. (2020). Tryptophan metabolism: A link between the gut microbiota and brain. *Advances in Nutrition (Bethesda, Md.)*, 11(3), 709–723. doi:10.1093/advances/nmz127

Harvard Health. (2021). Feed your gut. *Staying Healthy*. www.health.harvard.edu/staying-healthy/feed-your-gut

Holder, M. D. (2019). The contribution of food consumption to well-being. *Annals of Nutrition and Metabolism*, 74(suppl 2), 44–52. doi:10.1159/000499147

Yiengprugsawan, V., Banwell, C., Takeda, W., Dixon, J., Seubsman, S.-A., & Sleigh, A. C. (2015). Health, happiness and eating together: What can a large Thai cohort study tell us? *Global Journal of Health Science*, 7(4), 270–277. doi:10.5539/gjhs.v7n4p270

Zhong, B., Wang, X., & Yang, F. (2021). More than an apple: Better lunch enhances bus drivers' work performance and wellbeing. *International Journal of Occupational Safety and Ergonomics: JOSE*, 27(3), 874–883. https://doi-org.elib.tcd.ie/10.1080/10803548.2019.1662980

Play

Play is generally thought of as an activity for children, but adults can play too. Play is a self-directed and self-selected activity (Gray, 2009, 2013), so it is intrinsically motivated. Therefore, when playing, our actions should be purposeless, fun, and all-consuming, thus various activities can be considered play (Brown & Vaughan, 2009), for example:

1. Body play – jumping and moving around without a specific purpose; this includes rough-and-tumble activities
2. Object play – finding new and entertaining ways to use everyday objects; this includes using your imagination and pretend play
3. Social play – interacting with others in ways that are experimental and curious

The play draws on our imagination and engages our mind as active. At the same time, we do not experience distress when playing. There are some rules in play, but they are mostly implicit. For example, taking turns usually happens without explicit direction or arrangement. Play allows us to develop a sense of competency and control over our environment and helps us solve problems. Play helps us see other people's points of view and experience joy and creativity. Therefore, it is essential to cultivate play actively.

Research-based tools

Tool 33: Playlist (adapted from Frisch, 2006)

Write a list of activities you have enjoyed doing in the past or activities that you have heard other people doing. Don't think of how easy or difficult they are, just how much enjoyment you've had or could have from doing them. Also, bear in mind that active activities (e.g. jumping on a trampoline) can be more satisfying than passive activities (e.g. watching TV). Your list can include such activities as going to the cinema, listening to opera, visiting a museum, playing cards or board games, singing, dancing, going to a botanical garden, visiting a neighbour, sightseeing in the city, going to an antique sale, doing woodwork, hiking, bird watching, people-watching, bowling, reading do-it-yourself books, baking, scrapbooking, looking at pictures, cuddling, and many more. When creating your playlist, you can take time and keep adding to it for days or weeks.

Once you've listed your playful activities, develop a plan of what you can do every day over the next week to play. Then, try to follow your playful plan every day, even if it is just for 5 minutes

Please note that this tool was assessed as part of the quality-of-life therapy, not an individual intervention.

Tool 34: Stimulating playfulness (adapted from Proyer et al., 2021)

Over the next week, set aside 15 minutes before going to bed to reflect and write down one of the following:

1   Three playful things

   Write down three playful things you've experienced during the day. Also, consider who was involved in them and how you felt at the time.

2   Using playfulness

   Provide examples of how you have used your playfulness differently at work during the day. Also, write down who was involved in your playful experience and how you felt at the time.

3 Counting playfulness

Reflect on playful situations involving you or others during the day. Count how many individual, playful experiences you have witnessed.

Variation of practice

According to the OLIW-model, playfulness can take four different forms (Proyer, 2017):

1 Other-directed: we demonstrate playfulness while interacting with others to break conflict, tension, or routine.
2 Lighthearted, meaning we don't take life seriously, preferring to improvise rather than plan.
3 Intellectual, meaning we enjoy playing with complex ideas and enjoy the challenge of solving problems.
4 Whimsical, which indicates trying unchartered territory, dressing up, engaging with unusual activities.

To help you engage with play more, consider what type of playfulness suits you best and develop new ways of using your playfulness in daily life. Furthermore, sport is often considered a playful and beneficial activity for adults (Weldon et al., 2016). Try to approach the sport as a playground to promote physiological and additional mental health benefits. If we can access intrinsic motivation by making exercise enjoyable "vigorous play", we are more likely to adhere to exercise programmes and improve health outcomes (Biller, 2002). Using character strengths during exercise can make it a more playful activity (Hefferon & Mutrie, 2012); therefore, consider what strengths you can engage next time you exercise.

Check out other tools in this book

Try Humour tools, which can also help you play and provide you with extra energy.

Mental and physical health benefits

Stimulating playfulness has a short-term effect on wellbeing and reduction in symptoms of depression (Proyer et al., 2021). It predicts a range of positive outcomes as measured by PERMA Profiler, such as higher levels of positive emotions, lower levels of negative emotions, positive relationship, engagement, meaning, accomplishment, the decline in loneliness (Farley et al., 2021). Play is associated with an increased capacity for empathy and intimacy (Ward-Wimmer, 2003), improved creativity (Kets de Vries, 2012), cognition resulting in higher levels of academic achievement (Proyer, 2011), and improved ability to discover new coping strategies in the face of adversity (Proyer & Ruch, 2011). It provides opportunities for positive social interactions (Robinson et al., 2014). Given that playfulness is considered a positive emotion (Seligman et al., 2009), it has the impact of broadening and building our capacity to experience other positive emotions, encouraging an open mind and enhancing our resilience (Fredrickson, 1998).

A review of play interventions among clinical populations showed a range of positive outcomes in people with depression, anxiety, schizophrenia, and Asperger's syndrome (Berger et al., 2018). They included such outcomes as enhanced wellbeing, reduction of symptoms, and improvement in cognitive and affective functioning. Play is also effective as a coping strategy (Chang et al., 2013).

Playfulness in adults is associated with enhanced physical wellbeing and physical fitness (Proyer, 2013). Weldon et al. (2016) argue that adults can engage in various play-based activities to promote health and wellbeing. In a systemic review of the benefits of digital gaming in older adults, Hall et al. (2012) identified improvements in balance, strength, physical mobility, and reduction in pain as significant health benefits. A study on adults with type 1 diabetes showed that playing every day gave the participants a greater sense of coping with their chronic illness. Participants reported more positive mood, more remarkable ability to talk about their diabetes-related difficulties, and receiving more support (van Vleet et al., 2019). Thus, a playful approach to life and engaging in playful activities is not only fun but useful for our health and wellbeing.

Caveats

There is a danger that when you remember how good playing feels, you may become dissatisfied with your routinised work life and start to look for more opportunities to play in your work and other areas of your life (Brown & Vaughan, 2009). Also, beware of play that may cause harm to you or others. Too much risk can result in reckless behaviour.

References

Berger, P., Bitsch, F., Bröhl, H., & Falkenberg, I. (2018). Play and playfulness in psychiatry: A selective review. *International Journal of Play*, 7(2), 210–225. https://doi-org.elib.tcd.ie/10.1080/21594937.2017.1383341

Biller, H. B. (2002). *Creative fitness: Applying health psychology and exercise science to everyday life*. Greenwood Publishing Group.

Brown, S., & Vaughan, C. (2009). *Play: How it shapes the brain, opens the imagination and invigorates the soul*. Penguin.

Chang, P., Qian, X., & Yarnal, C. (2013). Using playfulness to cope with psychological stress: Taking into account both positive and negative emotions. *International Journal of Play*, 2(3), 273–296. doi:10.1080/21594937.2013.855414

Farley, A., Kennedy-Behr, A., & Brown, T. (2021). An investigation into the relationship between playfulness and well-being in Australian adults: An exploratory study. *OTJR: Occupation, Participation and Health*, 41(1), 56–64. https://doi.org/10.1177/1539449220945311

Fredrickson, B. L. (1998). What good are positive emotions? *Review of General Psychology*, 2, 300–319. doi:10.1037/ 1089-2680.2.3.300

Frisch, M. B. (2006). *Quality of life therapy: Applying a life satisfaction approach to positive psychology and cognitive therapy*. John Wiley & Sons Ltd.

Gray, P. (2009). Play as a foundation for hunter-gatherer social existence. *American Journal of Play*, 1, 476–522.

Gray, P. (2013). *Free to learn: Why unleashing the instinct to play will make our children happier, more self-reliant, and better prepared for life*. Basic Books.

Hall, A. K., Chavarria, E., Maneeratana, V., Chaney, B. H., & Bernhardt, J. M. (2012). Health benefits of digital videogames for older adults: A systematic review of the literature. *Games for Health: Research, Development, and Clinical Applications*, 1(6), 402–410.

Hefferon, K., & Mutrie, N. (2012). Physical activity as a 'stellar' positive psychology intervention. In E. Acevedo (Ed.), *Oxford Handbook of Exercise Psychology* (pp. 117–130). Oxford University Press.

Kets de Vries, M. F. R. (2012). Get back in the sandbox: Teaching CEOs how to play. *INSEAD Working Paper No. 2012/125/EFE*. http://dx.doi.org/10.2139/ssrn.2184916

Proyer, R. T. (2011). Being playful and smart? The relations of adult playfulness with psychometric and self-estimated intelligence and academic performance. *Learning and Individual Differences*, 21, 463–467. doi:10.1016/j.lindif.2011.02.003

Proyer, R. T. (2013). The wellbeing of playful adults: Adult playfulness, subjective wellbeing, physical wellbeing, and the pursuit of enjoyable activities. *European Journal of Humour Research*, 1, 84–98. doi:10.7592/EJHR2013.1.1.proyer

Proyer, R. T. (2017). A new structural model for the study of adult playfulness: Assessment and exploration of an understudied individual differences variable. *Personality and Individual Differences*, 108, 113–122. https://doi-org.elib.tcd.ie/10.1016/j.paid.2016.12.011

Proyer, R. T., Gander, F., Brauer, K., & Chick, G. (2021). Can playfulness be stimulated? A randomised placebo-controlled online playfulness intervention study on effects on trait playfulness, well-being, and depression. *Applied Psychology. Health and Well-Being, 13*(1), 129–151. https://doi-org.elib.tcd.ie/10.1111/aphw.12220

Proyer, R. T., & Ruch, W. (2011). The virtuousness of adult playfulness: The relation of playfulness with strengths of character. *Psychology of Well-Being: Theory, Research and Practice, 1,* 4. doi:10.1186/2211-1522-1-4

Robinson, L., Smith, M., & Segal, J. (2014). *Why play matters for adults.* www.helpguide.org/life/creative_play_fun_games.htm

Seligman, M. E. P., Ernst, R. M., Gillham, J., Reivich, K., & Linkins, M. (2009). Positive education: Positive psychology and classroom interventions. *Oxford Review of Education, 35,* 293–311.

Van Vleet, M., Helgeson, V. S., & Berg, C. A. (2019). The importance of having fun: Daily play among adults with type 1 diabetes. *Journal of Social and Personal Relationships, 36*(11–12), 3695–3710.

Ward-Wimmer, D. (2003). Introduction: The healing potential of adults at play. In C. E. Schaefer (Ed.), *Play therapy with adults* (pp. 1–11). Wiley and Sons Publisher.

Weldon, C., Baylis, D., & Tonkin, A. (2016). Lifestyle trends and their impact on health. In A. Tonkin & J. Whitaker (Eds.), *Play in healthcare: Using play to promote health and wellbeing across the adult lifespan* (pp. 85–98). Routledge.

Humour

When we think of humour, joy, laughter, and cheerfulness often come to mind. However, humour is a complex, multidimensional phenomenon comprising cognitive, emotional, and interpersonal components (Martin, 2007), and research on humour is nothing but serious. A sense of humour can be perceived as (1) an ability to amuse others, (2) tendency to laugh a lot and make jokes, (3) humorous temperament, (4) enjoyment of funny content, (5) a humorous attitude, (6) a particular world view, or (7) a coping strategy (Martin, 2003). The good news is that we can learn a sense of humour (Ruch & McGhee, 2014). Also, researchers tested humour tools as once-off interventions and more extended programmes; and both types were effective at enhancing participants' sense of humour.

Humour can be a shared social event between two or more people or an individual experience when it is an emotional response to a personal experience in one's day (Woodbury-Fariña & Antongiorgi, 2014). We can observe humour in others through playful verbal reactions, smiling, and laughter (Woodbury-Fariña & Antongiorgi, 2014).

Not all humour is good for us (Martin et al., 2003). The healthy types of humour are (1) affiliative humour, which is to make other people laugh, which results in group cohesiveness, and (2) self-enhancing humour, meaning that humour is used as a coping strategy when facing stress and adversity. These two types of humour have a robust adaptive effect and are therefore encouraged to use frequently. The unhealthy humour type which reduces our and other people's wellbeing is (3) aggressive humour, which includes sarcasm and ridiculing and manipulating others through humorous remarks; hence we should avoid it. The fourth type of humour, which reports lower levels of wellbeing than affiliative and self-enhancing humour, is (4) self-defeating humour associated with ill speaking of self about one's behaviour, characteristics, attitudes, outcomes. However, some researchers believe it is not too bad as long as this type of humour is associated with higher self-esteem, because using self-deprecation makes people less threatening to others, thus helping all parties build a stronger relationship (Heintz & Ruch, 2018).

Research-based tools

Tool 35: Three funny things (adapted from Gander et al., 2013)

Over the next week, set aside 15 minutes every evening and write down the three funniest things that have happened to you during the day. Reflect on the reasons those things happened and describe how they made you feel.

Tool 36: Counting funny things (adapted from Wellenzohn et al., 2016)

Every day over the next week, set aside 10 minutes and count any funny things you experienced during the day. Then reflect on the reasons those things happened to you.

Tool 37: Solving a stressful situation humorously (adapted from Wellenzohn et al., 2016)

Whenever you experience a stressful situation, afterwards, reflect on how it was and how you could have resolved it in a humorous way.

Tool 38: Applying humour (adapted from Wellenzohn et al., 2016)

At the end of the day, reflect on all the humorous situations you've experienced during the day and think of how you can build more humour into your next day by adding new activities that make you laugh.

Tool 39: Watching comedy (adapted from Mota Sousa et al., 2019)

Three or four times a week, over the next few weeks, watch your favourite comedy show on TV.

Tool 40: Laughter yoga (adapted from Yazdani et al., 2014)

Attend eight 1-hour sessions of laughter yoga. You may find it online, or you can join a group in your vicinity. In this experiment, participants had two sessions a week.

Tool 41: Seven humour habits programme (adapted from McGhee, 2010)

1. For a week, watch a range of comedy programmes and reflect on the type of sense of humour you have. Consider the strengths and weaknesses of your sense of humour.
2. Write down all the fun things you like doing, and make sure you plan to do two fun things each day for a week. Use props to get you in a fun mood, e.g. wearing a silly nose.
3. For a week, spend more time engaging in social laughter. Go to comedy clubs; watch comedy programmes or funny films. While watching funny programmes, try to laugh louder than usual. Also, when in stressful situations, force yourself to laugh and reflect on how it made you feel.
4. Every day for a week, spend a few minutes searching through funny phrases/puns in the newspapers, on notices, on the internet. Write them down to help you get into a habit of noticing them.
5. For a week, try to find something funny in your daily life. If you find it challenging to do, watch comedy programmes and reflect on similar incidents in your life.
6. Collect and learn some self-deprecating jokes.
7. List your usual daily hassles and reflect on how you can think of them differently if you adopt a lighter attitude towards them.

Please note that the effectiveness of this programme was assessed in its entirety as a facilitator-led programme, whereas we mentioned only selected aspects of it.

Mental and physical health benefits

Humour can be described as evoking the positive emotion of amusement (Ruch, 2001). There is also a positive thought process in remembering funny events. In addition, there is an attentional shift towards current positive thinking (Sanchez et al., 2014). This suggests that humour benefits us by building our cheerful emotional repertoire and opening our thought process to positive and expansive ways (Quoidbach et al., 2010; Fredrickson, 1998). In the workplace, affiliative and self-enhancing types of humour protect against burnout and are associated with higher work engagement (van den Broeck et al., 2012). In a 6-month follow-up study after a humour intervention, employees reported lower levels of stress and higher levels of work meaningfulness, work enjoyment, and flow experiences (Bartzik, 2021). Also, a meta-analysis of humour interventions showed that they significantly reduce symptoms of depression and anxiety and improve sleep quality (Zhao et al., 2019). As such, humour goes beyond the experiences of simple positive emotions.

Concerning physiological health, humour is associated with wound healing via increases in oxytocin levels, also responsible for bonding (Woodbury-Fariña & Antongiorgi, 2014). Furthermore, watching comedy during hemodialysis not only enhanced patients' sense of humour but also boosted their subjective wellbeing and decreased their symptoms of depression (Mota Sousa et al., 2019). Humour interventions are good not only for the patients but also their relatives, and caregivers in palliative care (Linge-Dahl et al., 2018). However, the results of the humour interventions for psychiatric patients are mixed.

Caveats

There is some evidence to suggest that humour interventions help reduce feelings of depression; however, more research is needed to assess if these gains are maintained over time (more than 6 months) (Wellenzohn et al., 2016). Also, be mindful of the type of humour you practice, as sarcastic and self-deprecating humour might not be effective in enhancing your or other people's wellbeing.

References

Bartzik, M., Bentrup, A., Hill, S., Bley, M., von Hirschhausen, E., Krause, G., Ahaus, P., Dahl-Dichmann, A., & Peifer, C. (2021). Care for joy: Evaluation of a humor intervention and its effects on stress, flow experience, work enjoyment, and meaningfulness of work. *Frontiers in Public Health, 9*, 667821. https://doi.org/10.3389/fpubh.2021.667821

den Broeck, A. V., Vander Elst, T., Dikkers, J., De Lange, A., & De Witte, H. (2012). This is funny: On the beneficial role of self-enhancing and affiliative humour in job design. *Psicothema, 24*(1), 87–93.

Fredrickson, B. L. (1998). What good are positive emotions? *Review of General Psychology, 2*, 300–319. doi:10.1037/ 1089–2680.2.3.300

Gander, F., Proyer, R. T., Ruch, W., & Wyss, T. (2013). Strength-based positive interventions: Further evidence for their potential in enhancing wellbeing and alleviating depression. *Journal of Happiness Studies, 14*, 1241–1259. doi:10.1007/s10902-012-9380-0

Heintz, S., & Ruch, W. (2018). Can self-defeating humor make you happy? Cognitive interviews reveal the adaptive side of the self-defeating humor style. *Humor, 31*(3), 451–472. https://doi.org/10.1515/humor-2017-0089

Linge-Dahl, L. M., Heintz, S., Ruch, W., & Radbruch, L. (2018). Humor assessment and interventions in palliative care: A systematic review. *Frontiers in Psychology, 9*. https://doi-org.elib.tcd.ie/10.3389/fpsyg.2018.00890

Martin, R. A. (2003). Sense of humor. In S. J. Lopez & C. R. Snyder (Eds.), *Positive psychological assessment: A handbook of models and measures*. American Psychological Association.

Martin, R. A. (2007). *The psychology of humor: An integrative approach*. Elsevier Science.

Martin, R. A., Puhlik-Doris, P., Larsen, G., Gray, J., & Weir, K. (2003). Individual differences in uses of humor and their relation to psychological well-being: Development of the humor styles questionnaire. *Journal of Research in Personality, 37*(1), 48–75. https://doi-org.elib.tcd.ie/10.1016/S0092-6566(02)00534-2

McGhee, P. E. (2010). *Humor as survival training for a stressed-out world: The 7 habits program*. Author House.

Mota Sousa, L. M., Antunes, A. V., Alves Marques-Vieira, C. M., Lopes Silva, P. C., Pedro Severino, S. S., & Guerreiro José, H. M. (2019). Effect of humor intervention on wellbeing, depression, and sense of humor in hemodialysis patients. *Enfermería Nefrológica, 22*(3), 256–265. https://doi-org.elib.tcd.ie/10.4321/S2254-28842019000300004

Quoidbach, J., Berry, E. V., Hansenne, M., & Mikolajczak, M. (2010). Positive emotion regulation and wellbeing: Comparing the impact of eight savoring and dampening strategies. *Personality and Individual Differences, 49*(5), 368–373. https://doi.org/10.1016/j.paid.2010.03.048

Ruch, W. (2001). The perception of humor. In A. W. Kaszniak (Ed.), *Emotions, qualia, and consciousness* (pp. 410–425). Word Scientific.

Ruch, W., & McGhee, P. E. (2014). Humor intervention programs. In A. C. Parks & S. M. Schueller (Eds.), *The Wiley Blackwell handbook of positive psychological interventions* (pp. 179–193). Wiley Blackwell. https://doi.org/10.1002/9781118315927.ch10

Sanchez, A., Vazquez, C., Gomez, D., & Joormann, J. (2014). Gaze-fixation to happy faces predicts mood repair after a negative mood induction. *Emotion, 14*(1), 85. https://doi.org/10.1037/a0034500

Wellenzohn, S., Proyer, R. T., & Ruch, W. (2016). Humor-based online positive psychology interventions: A randomized placebo-controlled long-term trial. *The Journal of Positive Psychology, 11*(6), 584–594. doi:10.1080/17439760.2015.1137624

Woodbury-Fariña, M. A., & Antongiorgi, J. L. (2014). Humor. *Psychiatric Clinics of North America, 37*(4), 561–578.

Yazdani, M., Esmaeilzadeh, M., Pahlavanzadeh, S., & Khaledi, F. (2014). The effect of laughter Yoga on general health among nursing students. *Iranian Journal of Nursing and Midwifery Research, 19*(1), 36–40.

Zhao, J., Yin, H., Zhang, G., Li, G., Shang, B., Wang, C., & Chen, L. (2019). A meta-analysis of randomized controlled trials of laughter and humour interventions on depression, anxiety and sleep quality in adults. *Journal of Advanced Nursing, 75*(11), 2435–2424.

Your reflection space

Which energising tools would you like to try? Why?
Which activities did you find most useful? How did you tweak them?

4 Coping tools

We face two types of challenges in life: daily hassles and traumas. Daily hassles describe the insistent stressors we try to cope with every day. For example, if you are a parent, it may be getting up early to get your children ready for school and realising that their uniforms are not clean – rushing to make everyone breakfast on time while dealing with a tantrum from a teenager and a 3-year-old at the same time or trying to cope with your daughter refusing to wear her tights and insisting she change them just as you were about to leave the house. And these are just the hassles that happen before 8:30 a.m.

Daily hassles can be copious, overwhelming, and relentless – people in their middle life experience more hassles than their younger or older counterparts (Burke, 2016). When we try to cope with daily hassles, we often feel exhausted, become irritable, and beat ourselves up for not being resilient enough. After all, everyone around us experiences them, and they seem okay. This is when we start wondering what is wrong with us, as hassles often make us feel bad about ourselves.

Traumas are different. They are serious events that occur in our lifetimes, such as the death of someone close to us, life-threatening illness, or a severe accident. There is a clear "before" and "after" relating to trauma; we remember our life before that horrible event happened to us and the aftermath. Traumas can take us a long time to recover from. Still, the good news is that most people bounce back after traumas, and only a small percentage experience Post-traumatic Stress Disorder (PTSD) or another negative consequence of it (Hefferon & Boniwell, 2011).

When it comes to the impact of daily hassles and traumas on our physical and physiological health, it is the relentless hassles that cause us more harm (see Burke, 2016 for a review). As such, they require us to keep practising our resilience day-in and day-out and improving our coping strategies, which is what this chapter is about.

DOI: 10.4324/9781003279594-6

Coping tools include:

1. Expressive writing
2. Optimism
3. Bibliotherapy
4. Stress mindset
5. Compassion

References

Burke, J. (2016). *Happiness after 30: The paradox of ageing*. Jumpp.

Hefferon, K., & Boniwell, I. (2011). *Positive psychology: Theory, research and applications*. Open University Press.

Expressive writing

I once worked with a client diagnosed with dyslexia (a learning difficulty affecting the acquisition of fluent and accurate reading and spelling skills). The thought of writing anything filled her with dread. Her automatic response was an absolute "No" when I told her about this tool. But then I shared with her a list of benefits for doing it, which were based on 30 years of rigorous research. Slowly, her reluctance turned into the willingness to try it and then enthusiasm after she experienced firsthand how useful it was, especially in situations when her worries kept her awake at night. Years later, she continued to use it. She spoke about this tool as a "pen friend", "her therapist", and "a helpful hand to figure out her worries and make life-decisions". Given that she found it helpful, perhaps so can you. After all, writing therapy is a long-standing clinical intervention (e.g. narrative exposure therapy, written exposure therapy, cognitive processing therapy, logotherapy, acceptance and commitment therapy) that has been recently tested for not only reducing illness but also enhancing wellbeing (Ruini & Mortara, 2021).

Research-based tools

Tool 42: The original expressive writing tool (adapted from Pennebaker, 1997)

Find a piece of paper and a pen. For the next 20 minutes, write about your deepest thoughts and feelings associated with your health. Repeat this activity every day for the next 3 to 5 days.

Tool 43: Book of life (adapted from Botella et al., 2017)

Another way of expressing self is by creating a Book of Life. This activity is a positive psychological twist on expressive writing and embracing technology at the same time. A Book of Life is a personal digital diary. It consists of several chapters and may include multimedia such as pictures, videos, art, music). Contribute to your Book of Life regularly with meaningful content, which includes all the good and bad events that happened in your life. Reflect on them and express them by writing *your* book of life.

Tool 44: Fairy tale writing (adapted from Masoni, 2019)

This is an emerging activity with limited research used with both adults and young people that encourages them to rewrite their stories by creating a narrative about their lives (Once upon a time, there was . . .). It is written as a third-person account (she/he) to help you distance yourself from your problems and view your challenges from a different perspective. When engaging in fairy tale writing, there are three steps you can follow: (1) identify your initial source of stress, (2) describe the journey of the protagonists with all the twists and turns they face, and (3) describe what your "happy ending" is or you expect it to be.

Variations of practice

Researchers found that hand-writing is more effective than typing (Brewin & Lennard, 1999). Also, if you're bilingual, you can express your thoughts in both languages, as it is more effective than forcing yourself to write in one (Youngsuk, 2008). When experiencing very traumatic events, it is sometimes easier for us to write in the third person (e.g. he did, she did); however, it is more effective to do it in the first person (e.g. I did) (Seih et al., 2011). This is why some therapists recommend starting with the third person if you struggle to express yourself and then moving towards the first-person writing.

If writing is not your thing, you can try to express yourself in other healthy ways, such as:

- Create music or art (see Feeling-good Tools for more detail)
- Create a vblog (without publishing it) to help you express yourself verbally if it is any easier.
- Use social media to express yourself by sharing thoughts and reflections about your life (Sauter, 2013)

- Use instant messaging with a professional (Hull et al., 2020) or friends.
- Use email to a professional or a friend to express yourself. For example, Sloan et al. (2015) introduced a concept of "therapy" that helps patients reduce symptoms of post-traumatic stress disorder by emailing a therapist twice a week for 10 weeks with their deepest thoughts and feelings.

Please note that there are differences in creative, expressive, and reflective writing (Lengelle et al., 2013). Expressive writing focuses on expressing your thoughts; reflective writing goes beyond expression into reflecting why something happened and considering an alternative response. If you want to take expression one step further, you may wish to combine reflective writing with expressive writing. Whilst expressive writing is about topics from your own life and events that happened to you, creative writing involves imagination and creativity and may not necessarily describe your life.

Mental and physical health benefits

The three main benefits that the expressive writing tool offers include physical functioning (e.g. improved immune system, reduction in doctors' visits, reducing pain), performance (e.g. improvement in grades in young people, lower incidents of absenteeism from work), and psychological (e.g. reduction in anxiety, depression, distress) (Kállay, 2015). However, while expressive writing is an effective tool for depression, it should not be used only as a once-off intervention (Reinhold et al., 2018). It is recommended that you engage with it regularly and write about specific challenges rather than generic ones. It is also a beneficial tool for individuals dealing with bereavement and grief (Range & Jenkins, 2010). Furthermore, if you have just retired, this tool may help you come to terms with life changes and enhance your wellbeing (Round & Burke, 2018). Thus, it is a useful tool for non-clinical populations.

Research with clinical patients shows mixed results. While it is effective for some mental disorders, such as PTSD (Qian et al., 2020), it is less effective in others. For example, a meta-analysis of research with breast cancer patients showed that expressive writing resulted in physical health improvement for up to 3 months after the intervention and some reduction of cancer symptoms; however, it showed no effect on psychological wellbeing or improvements in quality of life (Pok-Ja & Soo, 2016; Zachariae & O'Toole, 2015; Zhou et al., 2015). In addition, researchers found negligible benefits in people with advanced disease in palliative care (Kupeli et al., 2019). Therefore, you should use it with care.

Caveats

This activity is not effective for everyone. Some may gain more benefits from it than others. Also, when you're in a good mood, this activity may lower your mood. It is more effective when your mood is low and you want to figure out why and improve it. Also, if you experience any psychiatric conditions, it is recommended that you speak with a healthcare professional before engaging in this activity.

References

Botella, C., Banos, R. M., & Guillen, V. (2017). Positive technologies for improving health and well-being. In C. Proctor (Eds.), *Positive Psychology Interventions in Practice*. Springer, Cham. https://doi.org/10.1007/978-3-319-51787-2_13

Brewin, C. R., & Lennard, H. (1999). Effects of mode of writing on emotional narratives. *Journal of Traumatic Stress, 12*(2), 355. https://doi-org.elib.tcd.ie/10.1023/A:1024736828322

Hull, T. D., Malgaroli, M., Connolly, P. S., Feuerstein, S., & Simon, N. M. (2020). Two-way messaging therapy for depression and anxiety: Longitudinal response trajectories. *BMC Psychiatry, 20*(1), 1–12. https://doi-org.elib.tcd.ie/10.1186/s12888-020-02721-x

Kállay, É. (2015). Physical and psychological benefits of written emotional expression: Review of meta-analyses and recommendations. *European Psychologist, 20*(4), 242–251. https://doi-org.elib.tcd.ie/10.1027/1016-9040/a000231

Kim, Y. (2008). Effects of expressive writing among bilinguals: Exploring psychological wellbeing and social behaviour. *British Journal of Health Psychology, 13*(Pt 1), 43–47. https://doi.org/10.1348/135910707X251225

Kupeli, N., Chatzitheodorou, G., Troop, N. A., McInnerney, D., Stone, P., & Candy, B. (2019). Expressive writing as a therapeutic intervention for people with advanced disease: A systematic review. *BMC Palliative Care, 18*(1), N.PAG. https://doi-org.elib.tcd.ie/10.1186/s12904-019-0449-y

Lengelle, R., Meijers, F., Poell, R., & Post, M. (2013). The effects of creative, expressive, and reflective writing on career learning: An explorative study. *Journal of Vocational Behavior, 83*(3), 419–427. https://doi-org.elib.tcd.ie/10.1016/j.jvb.2013.06.014

Masoni, L. (2019). *Tale, performance, and culture in EFL storytelling with young learners: Stories meant to be told*. Cambridge Scholars Publishing.

Pennebaker, J. W. (1997). Writing about emotional experiences as a therapeutic process. *Psychological Science, 8*, 162–166.

Pok-Ja Oh, & Soo Hyun Kim. (2016). The effects of expressive writing interventions for patients with cancer: A meta-analysis. *Oncology Nursing Forum, 43*(4), 468–479. https://doi-org.elib.tcd.ie/10.1188/16.ONF.468-479

Qian, J., Zhou, X., Sun, X., Wu, M., Sun, S., & Yu, X. (2020). Effects of expressive writing intervention for women's PTSD, depression, anxiety and stress related to pregnancy: A meta-analysis of randomized controlled trials. *Psychiatry Research, 288*, 112933. https://doi-org.elib.tcd.ie/10.1016/j.psychres.2020.112933

Range, L., & Jenkins, S. R. (2010). Who benefits from Pennebaker's expressive writing? Research recommendations from three ender theories. *Sex Roles, 63*, 149–163.

Reinhold, M., Bürkner, P., & Holling, H. (2018). Effects of expressive writing on depressive symptoms – A meta-analysis. *Clinical Psychology: Science and Practice, 25*(1). https://doi-org.elib.tcd.ie/10.1037/h0101749

Round, J., & Burke, J. (2018). A dream of a retirement: The longitudinal experiences and perceived retirement wellbeing of recent retirees following a tailored intervention linking best possible self-expressive writing with goal-setting. *International Coaching Psychology Review, 13*(2), 27–45.

Ruini, C., & Mortara, C. C. (2021). Writing technique across psychotherapies – from traditional expressive writing to new positive psychology interventions: A narrative review. *Journal of Contemporary Psychotherapy*. https://doi.org/10.1007/s10879-021-09520-9

Sauter, T. (2013). 'What's on your mind?' Writing on Facebook as a tool for self-formation. *New Media & Society, 16*(5), 823–839.

Seih, Y.-T., Chung, C., & Pennebaker, J. (2011). Experimental manipulations of perspective taking and perspective switching in expressive writing. *Cognition & Emotion, 25*(5), 926–938. https://doi-org.elib.tcd.ie/10.1080/02699931.2010.512123

Sloan, D. M., Sawyer, A. T., Lowmaster, S. E., Wernick, J., & Marx, B. P. (2015). Efficacy of narrative writing as an intervention for PTSD: Does the evidence support its use? *Journal of Contemporary Psychotherapy, 45*(4), 215–225.

Youngsuk, K. (2008) Effects of expressive writing among bilinguals: Exploring psychological well-being and social behaviour. *British Journal of Health Psychology, 13*, 43–47.

Zachariae, R., & O'Toole, M. S. (2015). The effect of expressive writing intervention on psychological and physical health outcomes in cancer patients – a systematic review and meta-analysis. *Psycho-Oncology, 24*(11), 1349–1359. https://doi-org.elib.tcd.ie/10.1002/pon.3802

Zhou, C., Wu, Y., An, S., & Li, X. (2015). Effect of expressive writing intervention on health outcomes in breast cancer patients: A systematic review and meta-analysis of randomized controlled trials. *PLoS One, 10*(7), 1–19. https://doi-org.elib.tcd.ie/10.1371/journal.pone.0131802

Optimism

Most people are optimistic because our brain generates an optimism bias that helps us keep going and expect the best from life (Sharot et al.,

2007). For example, we expect to live longer than others, be happier than an average person, and avoid adversity such as divorce when we get married. Even when faced with hard facts that should logically challenge our optimistic beliefs, our brain counteracts them, and we choose positive illusion over uncomfortable reality (Sharot et al., 2011). This optimistic bias increases as we age (Chowdhury et al., 2014), making us most optimistic in our older days.

There are essentially two approaches to optimism, one of which sees it as a personality trait and the other as a way of thinking. The latter approach, exemplified by the psychologist Martin Seligman, has produced promising evidence showing that optimism can be learned. For Seligman (1998), optimism is how you think about setbacks and victories. Optimistic people, when they have a setback, believe that:

1   It's temporary.
2   They can change it.
3   It's just this one situation.

Pessimistic people believe that:

1   It's going to last forever.
2   They cannot change it.
3   It's going to undermine everything they do.

Conversely, when a good thing happens, the optimistic people think:

1   It's going to last forever.
2   They made it happen.
3   It's going to help them in every life circumstance.

When good things happen to the pessimistic people, they think:

1   It's just this one situation.
2   I didn't do it.
3   It's just going to help me in this one domain I'm in.

The key idea here is that our feelings of optimism or pessimism depend not on the events themselves but on how we characteristically think about them – and that's something we can change.

Research-based tools

Tool 45: ABCD analysis (Seligman, 1998)

During the next week, each day, think about a situation you found difficult or stressful using the following headings:

- **A** = **Adversity** or **A**ntecedent event you found difficult: be objective about the situation and record your description of what happened, not your evaluation of it.
- **B** = your **Beliefs** about the situation or event: record how you interpreted the event; how did you explain it to yourself?
- **C** – **Consequences**: record what you felt and what you did.

When you identify your beliefs and recognise their effects on your emotions and behaviours, you can change them to more positive thought patterns by using distraction, distancing, and disputation.

1. **Distract** involves doing something to change the focus of your attention. Simple distraction techniques include saying STOP and hitting the table; snapping your wrist with a rubber band; looking at a flashcard with STOP written on it; writing down your pessimistic ruminations immediately; postponing rumination until a later time and for a set period.
2. **Distance** involves telling yourself that your beliefs are just that: beliefs. Your pessimistic interpretation of the situation is just one set of beliefs – there are always more optimistic explanations, some of which may be equally valid.
3. **Dispute** involves asking yourself what evidence there is for your beliefs and whether the evidence supports your beliefs. Are there an alternative, more optimistic ways of looking at the situation? Even if your belief is correct, you can reduce its impact by asking what the real implications are: catastrophe or a bit of a temporary nuisance? Finally, ask yourself which set of beliefs is most useful for you to improve your mood and achieve your goals.

Please note this activity has been validated as part of the Penn Resiliency Programme (Gillham & Reivich, 2004), not on its own. It is also an integral part of the cognitive behavioural therapy approach (Ellis, 1962).

Variations of practice

Carr (2020) provides additional practical methods that help the ABC identification process. The first is Socratic questioning, which you can use to dispute pessimistic beliefs. Examples include questions such as: Have I any evidence against my belief? Are there any facts about the situation that I am discounting? What questions would I ask my closest friend who expressed such a view? Am I blaming myself for something that I couldn't control? The second technique is conducting behavioural experiments to provide evidence to test your pessimistic belief. For example, suppose you failed at a particular task because you are "stupid and useless at everything". In that case, you might set yourself a moderately challenging task and notice that you can complete it competently.

A meta-analysis of psychological interventions aiming to enhance optimism recommended a range of tools discussed in this book, such as Best Possible Self tools, Looking Forward to Tomorrow tool, and Self-Compassion tool (Malouff & Schutte, 2017).

Mental and physical health benefits

Optimism is associated with less distress when dealing with problems, better adaptation to adverse events, less depression and anxiety, more significant effort to solve problems and better use of problem-focused coping, better success in school, in sports, at work, in politics and personal relationships (Boniwell & Tunariu, 2019; Carver et al., 2010; Peterson et al., 2012). Substantial research has also demonstrated a significant predictive relationship between optimism and a range of physical outcomes, including immune functioning, cardiovascular disease risk and mortality, cancer outcomes, outcomes related to pregnancy, physical symptoms, and pain (Rasmussen et al., 2009; Rozanski et al., 2019). In addition, optimists have longer telomeres than pessimists, and the length of telomeres is associated with stress and ageing; thus, optimistic thinking is beneficial in sustaining cellular health (Schutte & Malouff, 2020). The predictive relationship between optimism and longevity is particularly noteworthy, with optimists having a 30% lower chance of coronary-related death over eight years, which suggests that promotion of optimism and reduction in pessimism may be necessary for preventive health (Rozanski et al., 2019; Tindle et al., 2012). Thus, even though thinking optimistically might not be natural to you, it is worthwhile giving it a try, especially to help you find the motivation to keep pursuing a goal.

Caveats

Engaging in blind unrealistic optimism may be unhealthy for long-term physical and psychological wellbeing. Introducing *positive realism* or *flexible optimism* into our thinking means that we can avoid "wishful thinking" (Boniwell & Tunariu, 2019). A pessimistic thinking style can be helpful in certain high-risk situations, such as those in which the cost of failure is remarkably high. Examples include a significant business decision or a personal financial decision. Here, it is prudent to plan for the worst-case scenario. You can, of course, hope for the best, like an optimist (Norem & Chang, 2002; Carr, 2020)! Also, according to the theory of defensive pessimism, being optimistic may cause some people anxiety, as they need to consider the worst-case scenario when faced with a challenge (Norem, 2001). As they start practising optimism without reflecting on what can go wrong and finding strategies for it, they become even more anxious. Whilst usually, pessimism leads to withdrawal and failure in accomplishing a goal, optimism and defensive pessimism lead to success. Nonetheless, the defensive pessimism paradigm was challenged by Araki (2012), who claimed that some of the characteristics of defensive pessimists were attributed to strategic optimists; hence the researcher questioned its validity. Future research will hopefully explore this topic further.

References

Araki, Y. (2012). Experimental investigation of defensive pessimism and learned helplessness. *Japanese Journal of Health Psychology, 25*(1), 104–113. https://doi-org.elib.tcd.ie/10.11560/jahp.25.1_104

Boniwell, I., & Tunariu, A. D. (2019). *Positive psychology: Theory, research and applications.* (2nd ed.). McGraw Hill Open University Press.

Carr, A. (2020). *Positive psychology and you: A self-development guide.* Routledge.

Carver, C. S., Scheier, M. F., & Segerstrom, S. C. (2010). Optimism. *Clinical Psychology Review, 30,* 879–889. doi:10.1016/j.cpr.2010.01.006

Chowdhury, R., Sharot, T., Wolfe, T., Düzel, E., & Dolan, R. J. (2014). Optimistic update bias increases in older age. *Psychological Medicine, 44*(9), 2003–2012. https://doi-org.elib.tcd.ie/10.1017/S0033291713002602

Ellis, A. (1962). *Reason and emotion in psychotherapy.* Lyle Stuart.

Gillham, J., & Reivich, K. (2004). Cultivating optimism in childhood and adolescence. *Annals of the American Academy of Political & Social Science, 591,* 146–163. https://doi-org.elib.tcd.ie/10.1177/0002716203260095

Malouff, J. M., & Schutte, N. S. (2017). Can psychological interventions increase optimism? A meta-analysis. *The Journal of Positive Psychology, 12*(6), 594–604. https://doi-org.elib.tcd.ie/10.1080/17439760.201

Norem, J. K. (2001). *The positive power of negative thinking: Using defensive pessimism to manage anxiety and perform at your peak.* Basic Books.

Norem, J. K., & Chang, E. C. (2002). The positive psychology of negative thinking. *Journal of Clinical Psychology, 58*(9), 993–1001.

Peterson, P., Park, N., & Kim, E. S. (2012). Can optimism decrease the risk of illness and disease among the elderly? *Aging Health, 8*(1), 5–8. doi:10.2217/ahe.11.81

Rasmussen, H. N., Scheier, M. F., & Greenhouse, J. B. (2009). Optimism and physical health: A meta-analytic review. *Annals of Behavioral Medicine*, *37*(3), 239–256. doi:10.1007/s12160-009-9111-x

Rozanski, A., Bavishi, C., Kubzansky, L. D., & Cohen, M. D. (2019). Association of optimism with cardiovascular events and all-cause mortality. A systematic review and meta-analysis. *JAMA Network Open*, *2*(9), 10.1001/jamanetworkopen.2019.12200

Schutte, N., & Malouff, J. M. (2022). The association between optimism and telomere length: A meta-analysis. *The Journal of Positive Psychology*, *17*(1), 82–88. doi:10.1080/17439760.2020.1832249

Seligman, M. E. P. (1998). *Learned optimism: How to change your mind and your life.* Free Press.

Sharot, T., Korn, C. W., & Dolan, R. J. (2011). How unrealistic optimism is maintained in the face of reality. *Nature Neuroscience*, *14*(11), 1475–1479. https://doi-org.elib.tcd.ie/10.1038/nn.2949

Sharot, T., Riccardi, A. M., Raio, C. M., & Phelps, E. A. (2007). Neural mechanisms mediating optimism bias. *Nature*, *450*(7166), 102–105. https://doi-org.elib.tcd.ie/10.1038/nature06280

Tindle, H., Belnap, B. H., Houck, P. R., Mazumdar, S., Scheier, M. F., & Rollman, B. L. (2012). Optimism, response to treatment of depression, and re-hospitalization after coronary artery bypass graft surgery. *Psychosomatic Medicine*, *74*(2), 200–207.

Bibliotherapy

In the last decade, the self-help industry has grown exponentially, and its annual turnover is now more than 10 billion euros. The self-help titles crowd the top 10 lists of best-selling books each month, with millions of people reading and listening to them daily. On the one hand, the interest in self-help books highlights the health challenges that so many of us seem to experience nowadays, which drive us towards the self-help industry; on the other hand, it points to the books helping people to enhance their health and wellbeing. Otherwise, why else would they read them?

Bibliotherapy, otherwise known as literature or library therapy, refers to a technique of using books and multimedia to enhance health and wellbeing in the following contexts: (1) clinical settings, e.g. guiding readers through a cognitive behavioural therapy (CBT) treatment process to reduce their depression; (2) developmental bibliotherapy to provide clients with information and advice on how to cope with various situations, and is used as a preventative measure to experiencing health issues, e.g. guiding readers through potential pitfalls after their cancer diagnosis or advising them about activities they can do to enhance their wellbeing and prevent illness; (3) creative, using poetry, or fiction writing to analyse thoughts and feelings (Sevinç, 2019). Bibliotherapy is often used in conjunction with therapy, allowing individuals to take control of their choices, thoughts, and feelings in a safe environment. Books can also be used to guide readers through life challenges they have never experienced and provide them with informed advice on how to do it on their own. For example, we may read a book about grief after someone close to us dies to help us make sense of the sadness and emptiness we experience. Alternatively, we may read a book about someone's journey to enhanced wellbeing and take some direct or indirect advice as to what changes we could make in our lives to improve our quality of life.

Research-based tools

Tool 46: Read and practice tools in a self-help book (adapted from Wimberley et al., 2016)

Select a self-help book that helps you develop knowledge and skills in an area you are interested in. It can be how to cope with grief, enhance wellbeing, and accomplish whatever you wish to accomplish. Ensure that the self-help book you select is written by an academic or someone with expertise in this area. Also, check if the book has tools or activities that you can complete to practice your skills. For example, in the original experiment, the book was *Present Perfect*, written by Pavel Somov (2010). Readers were invited to stop and engage in mindfulness practice, which was described in detail. They were asked to read it daily and stop to engage in practice. This approach to bibliotherapy resulted in a range of positive outcomes.

Tool 47: Join a book club (adapted from Pettersson, 2016)

Join a regular club or gathering in your geographical area the objective of which is to read books and discuss them.

Tool 48: Read fiction (adapted from Kidd & Castano, 2013)

If you enjoy reading, make sure you read fiction books regularly. Now and then, allow yourself to block out a more significant amount of time to immerse yourself further into the stories.

Variations of practice

Apart from bibliotherapy, you may also consider cinematherapy, whereby you watch films to help you reflect upon life and provide you with advice on what you can do to enhance your wellbeing.

Mental and physical health benefits

Reading books, as opposed to newspapers or magazines or not reading at all, is associated with a 2-year reduction in mortality (Bavishi et al., 2016). It significantly boosts our brain cell connectivity, helping us, especially on the days when we finish a book or become engrossed in it, to think more clearly (Berns et al., 2013). It is also one of the most effective ways to reduce stress and improve our empathy (Mar et al., 2009). Moreover, reading a book before going to bed improves sleep quality (Finucane et al., 2021). However, it is better to opt for a printed book than a digital one, as digital books decrease sleepiness by approximately 30 minutes (Grønli et al., 2016), although there is no evidence to suggest they impact sleep quality or length.

Furthermore, specific self-help books help us develop our knowledge and skills, contributing to psychological changes. For example, reading a book about self-esteem enhanced participants' general, family, professional, and total self-esteem (Salimi et al., 2014). Reading a book about health anxiety reduced patients' anxiety about their health. It reassured them compared to a group who had not undergone bibliotherapy and only participated in hospital visits, discussing their worries with medical professionals (Jones, 2002). Organising a book club for the elderly who experienced mild dementia resulted in improvements in functional, cognitive, and emotional, not to mention the social components of wellbeing (Rotenberg-Shpigelman & Maeir, 2011). Researchers noted similar results among individuals with intellectual disabilities (Hollins et al., 2016).

A meta-analysis of studies with almost a thousand participants identified that bibliotherapy was effective in reducing symptoms of depression and anxiety (Yuan et al., 2018). Specifically, reading a research-based positive psychology self-help book (as an alternative to the majority of the books based on cognitive behaviour therapy) and completing activities associated with it over 8 weeks resulted in participants' decrease of depression and increase of wellbeing (Hanson, 2019). Therefore, regardless if it is a book of fiction or a self-help book, bibliotherapy may help you enhance your wellbeing.

Caveat

Given that the publishing market is saturated with self-help books including many self-published books, it is important to discern the authors' credentials before you read the book and follow their advice.

References

Bavishi, A., Slade, M. D., & Levy, B. R. (2016). A chapter a day: Association of book reading with longevity. *Social Science & Medicine (1982)*, 164, 44–48. https://doi.org/10.1016/j.socscimed.2016.07.014

Berns, G. S., Blaine, K., Prietula, M. J., & Pye, B. E. (2013). Short- and long-term effects of a novel on connectivity in the brain. *Brain Connectivity*, 3(6), 590–600. https://doi-org.elib.tcd.ie/10.1089/brain.2013.0166

Finucane, E., O'Brien, A., Treweek, S., Newell, J., Das, K., Chapman, S., Wicks, P., Galvin, S., Healy, P., Biesty, L., Gillies, K., Noel-Storr, A., Gardner, H., O'Reilly, M. F., & Devane, D. (2021). Does reading a book in bed make a difference to sleep in comparison to not reading a book in bed? The People's Trial-an online, pragmatic, randomised trial. *Trials*, 22(1), 873. https://doi-org.elib.tcd.ie/10.1186/s13063-021-05831-3

Grønli, J., Byrkjedal, I. K., Bjorvatn, B., Nødtvedt, Ø., Hamre, B., & Pallesen, S. (2016). Reading from an iPad or from a book in bed: The impact on human sleep. A randomized controlled crossover trial. *Sleep Medicine*, 21, 86–92. https://doi-org.elib.tcd.ie/10.1016/j.sleep.2016.02.006

Hanson, K. (2019). Positive psychology for overcoming symptoms of depression: A pilot study exploring the efficacy of a positive psychology self-help book versus a CBT self-help book. *Behavioural & Cognitive Psychotherapy*, 47(1), 95–113. https://doi-org.elib.tcd.ie/10.1017/S1352465818000218

Hollins, S., Egerton, J., & Carpenter, B. (2016). Book clubs for people with intellectual disabilities: The evidence and impact on wellbeing and community participation of reading wordless books. *Advances in Mental Health & Intellectual Disabilities*, 10(5), 275–283. https://doi-org.elib.tcd.ie/10.1108/AMHID-08-2016-0020

Jones, F. A. (2002). The role of bibliotherapy in health anxiety: An experimental study. *British Journal of Community Nursing*, 7(10), 498–504. https://doi-org.elib.tcd.ie/10.12968/bjcn.2002.7.10.10662

Kidd, D. C., & Castano, E. (2013). Reading literary fiction improves theory of mind. *Science*, 342(6156), 377–380. https://doi.org/10.1126/science.1239918

Mar, R. A., Oatley, K., & Peterson, J. B. (2009). Exploring the link between reading fiction and empathy: Ruling out individual differences and examining outcomes. *Communications: The European Journal of Communication Research*, 34(4), 407–428. https://doi-org.elib.tcd.ie/10.1515/comm.2009.025

Rotenberg-Shpigelman, S., & Maeir, A. (2011). Participation-centered treatment for elderly with mild cognitive deficits: A "book club" group case study. *Physical & Occupational Therapy in Geriatrics*, 29(3), 222–232. https://doi-org.elib.tcd.ie/10.3109/02703181.2011.604149

Salimi, S., Zare-Farashbandi, F., Papi, A., Samouei, R., & Hassanzadeh, A. (2014). The effect of group bibliotherapy on the self-esteem of female students living in dormitory. *Journal of Education and Health Promotion*, 3, 89. https://doi-org.elib.tcd.ie/10.4103/2277-9531.139643

Sevinç, G. (2019). Healing mental health through reading: Bibliotherapy. *Current Approaches in Psychiatry/Psikiyatride Guncel Yaklasimlar*, 11(4), 483–495. https://doi-org.elib.tcd.ie/10.18863/pgy.474083

Wimberley, T. E., Mintz, L. B., & Suh, H. (2016). Perfectionism and mindfulness: Effectiveness of a bibliotherapy intervention. *Mindfulness*, 7(2), 433–444. https://doi-org.elib.tcd.ie/10.1007/s12671-015-0460-1

Yuan, S., Zhou, X., Zhang, Y., Zhang, H., Pu, J., Yang, L., Liu, L., Jiang, X., & Xie, P. (2018). Comparative efficacy and acceptability of bibliotherapy for depression and anxiety disorders in children and adolescents: A meta-analysis of randomized clinical trials. *Neuropsychiatric Disease and Treatment*, 14, 353–365. https://doi.org/10.2147/NDT.S152747

Stress mindset

As we go about our daily lives, we are continually exposed to enormous quantities of information. To manage this, we need a simplified system, a set of mental lenses to filter information about the world and ourselves. These lenses are called mindsets, and there is increasing evidence that the mindsets we adopt have profound effects on our physiology, our behaviour, and even our life spans (Crum et al., 2011; Dweck, 2017; Pagnini et al., 2019; Seligman, 1998). This can be seen, for example, in the placebo effect, in which an inert substance can cause a marked physiological response depending on the recipient's mindset (Price et al., 2008).

This increased understanding of the power of mindsets has now been used to alter the effects of stress. But unfortunately, most of us see stress as something negative, something to be avoided. While there is indeed a significant body of research demonstrating the negative impact of stress, significantly prolonged stress, on our mental and physical health (e.g. Yaribeygi et al., 2017; Schneiderman et al., 2005), new research is showing that stress can be good for us and that we can use it to enhance our performance.

It is important to note how we evolved as a species before considering a typically stressful situation for the average person in the 21st century. Although we have evolved into conscious, rational creatures with a high degree of brainpower compared to other members of the animal kingdom, we are still mammals. As mammals, we have a finely tuned fight-or-flight response to help protect us in the wild. When our ancestors were subsisting in the great ancient forests of the world, they did not have the luxury of considering whether a rattling bush was the wind or a predator. They ran. At that moment, several things must happen within nanoseconds[1] to prepare the body to flee or stay and fight. As non-predators, we usually ran.

To run, you need energy, and that energy comes from fat and sugars stored throughout the body, especially sugars stored in the liver (glycogen).

We need oxygen to help our muscles work faster to help us run. Therefore, our hearts beat faster, blood pressure rises, and breathing increases. We have no time to digest food, so digestion stops, and appetites are put on the back burner. Our pupils dilate to pick up peripheral movement. Our eardrums re-focus from human conversation frequencies to the low rumble of predators and the high pitch of prey being attacked. Libido diminishes immediately, and we develop a tunnel vision–like focus in which we only have one mission – escape. Sweating increases, and this is believed to signal to fellow prey that something dangerous is happening (they smell it). The immune system becomes activated to prepare for a bite. Predators' mouths contain billions of bacteria that can cause infection. A ready immune response can help fight that infection immediately. Assuming our ancestors outran the predator, all systems would return to a balanced state, and the individual mammal would get on with their foraging or other tasks.

However, if this ancestor was bitten but managed to escape to their cave, they would experience sickness behaviour. In sickness behaviour, we become anti-social and fatigued (we want to sleep in the safety of a dark cave). We have no appetite or libido, and we usually have an activated immune system that increases our temperature to fight infection. These characteristics help keep us safe from predators and prevent us from infecting the tribe (if a transmissible disease causes an infection). When the infection subsides, we become more social and re-engage with life. It is worth bearing in mind that stress in the modern world can also induce sickness behaviour in the absence of a bite from a predator or infection. Have you ever experienced the symptoms of sickness behaviour because of difficulties in the workplace or the home?

When you experience a stressful situation, say someone challenges you at work, the liver dumps fat and sugar into your bloodstream to give you fuel and that extra energy. Your breathing increases and deepens to help you take in more oxygen to feed your muscles and organs. Your heart rate speeds up to deliver oxygen, fat, and sugar to your muscles and organs to help you cope more effectively with this challenging situation. You also have a cocktail of chemicals rapidly spreading in your body, such as endorphins, adrenaline, testosterone, and dopamine. You are now experiencing a stressful episode, your is heart pounding, the tips of your fingers may be tingling, and you feel powerful energy within you. It is your body helping you to cope with this situation effectively. You need this oxygen delivered to your brain to think faster and find a better solution for dealing with the challenge you are facing. You need the fat and sugar in your muscles to run away from the situation if it is dangerous. You need adrenaline to help activate your resources.

What your body expects you to do with this excess energy is to use it wisely and resolve the issue or the challenge you are facing as soon as possible. It provides you with all the resources in its power to help you do it. However, what sometimes happens is that we ignore our bodies and do very little or nothing. When we do nothing and pretend that the problem does not exist (denial), our thoughts disengage from the issue. Still, our body gets us ready to tackle the problem as our subconscious alerts us that it is unresolved. In other words, we continue to experience the symptoms of stress, except it no longer happens at work but at home, when we sit with our family and cannot switch off; then later at night, when we wake up at 3 a.m. for no apparent reason. The longer this state continues, the more we start experiencing distress. It is a distress that is harmful to us, not stress. Stress helps, not hinders us.

The key idea is that our mindset when dealing with stress significantly affects our select coping strategies. When we adopt a stress-is-debilitating mindset, we tend to use less effective coping strategies when faced with stress, such as denial; whereas when we have stressed-is-enhancing mindset, we tend to feel the stress in our body (embodiment), stop and assess why we feel stress (find the underlying cause of what is the source of stress), use our resources to take steps to resolve it (get help, produce an action plan), or tackle it head-on (Crum et al., 2013). When we approach our stressful situations with the stress-is-enhancing mindset, our stress supports us in improving our performance, productivity, and health; and the stress-is-debilitating mindset results in debilitating consequences for these outcomes.

Recently, researchers proposed that apart from these dichotomous mindsets, many people report having a mixed mindset, whereby in some situations, they practice the stress-is-enhancing mindset, and in other situations, the stress-is-debilitating mindset (O'Hare & Burke, forthcoming). For example, you may be great at dealing with stress at work and tend to have a stress-is-enhancing attitude towards the stress you experience at work; however, your attitude doesn't hold for your personal life, where you mostly have a stress-is-debilitating mindset. Other researchers differentiated between generic attitude toward stress and specific situations that affect our mindsets (Jenkins et al., 2021). For example, you may hold a belief that stress is bad, but when asked how you coped with a specific stressful event, you may have a stress-is-enhancing mindset that allows you to summon your resources to cope with stressful events. Therefore, much more research is required to identify the nuances of stress mindset.

In the meantime, however, the good news is that you can change the stress mindset, which impacts our psychological (Burke, 2018; Crum et al., 2013, 2017) as well as physiological resources (Park et al., 2018).

An online educational intervention showed changes in brain waves, measured by EEG, confirming that learning about the positive effects of stress reduces the adverse effects of stress (Park et al., 2018). Activities in this section will help you do it.

Research-based tools

Tool 49: Stanford Lab (Crum et al., 2022)

Alia Crum and colleagues at the Stanford Mind and Body Lab have developed a method to change your stress mindset and embrace a more positive one. You can access the entire method for rethinking stress at https://mbl.stanford.edu/interventions-toolkits/rethink-stress-intervention.

Essentially, the method involves three phases:

1 Acknowledge your stress: What is stressing you right now, and how do you typically react mentally and physically and in terms of your behaviour?
2 Welcome your stress: we only get stressed when we care about something, our positive purpose. What is it that you care about (motivation or a personal value) that makes you stressed?
3 Use your stress: considering what you discovered in Step 2 about your positive purpose, and ask yourself if your typical reactions are helping or hindering your purpose and how you can make them enhance.

Variations in practice

One of our clients adopted a new ritual in his stressful life. Given that work was his most significant source of stress, before leaving the office, he wrote down a list of causes of his stress. While driving home, he was reflecting on what he could have done differently (what he had learnt) and how to reduce the impact of this stressor the next day. By the time he got home, he had a few ideas about it and scribbled them down in his notepad before putting the notepad into his glovebox and walking through the front door. This way, he could leave the work behind, as he spent relaxing time with his family. This simple reflection activity made a significant difference in his life. A year later, he talked about his work with joy and no longer considered it stressful. His stress mindset had altered, and a more effective coping strategy replaced his denial. This technique has worked for him, it may also work for you.

Whereas research cited here has provided empirical evidence for the importance of mindsets, there is a long history in philosophy and literature of such approaches. Particularly worth reading in this context are *Meditations* by the Roman emperor Marcus Aurelius (2002) and *Man's Search for Meaning* by Victor Frankl (1959). In addition, a brief questionnaire, the Stress Mindset Measure, for adults allows you to assess the degree to which you possess a "stress is enhancing" mindset (Crum et al., 2013). There is also a version for young people (Park et al., 2018).

Several experimental studies helped participants successfully adapt their stress-is-enhancing mindset. For example, Burke (2018) designed a 3-hour training session attended by over 900 people, the main components of which included stress-education and cognitive behavioural therapy methods to help participants challenge their negative beliefs about stress. Keech and colleagues (2021) used mental imagery to change students' stress mindset. Also, Maarsingh et al. (2019) used an innovative method of a virtual reality game that applied biofeedback. While all these interventions showed evidence of enhancing participants' stress mindset, the process involved was longer than a self-administered tool, which is why it is not mentioned as one of the tools. What all these studies had in common was their educational component that helped participants understand the positive effects of stress. Thus, if you wish to remind yourself about it in the future, we encourage you to read the introduction to this section once again and search for additional articles online about the benefits of stress. It may help you enhance your stress mindset and engage in more effective coping strategies.

Check out other tools in this book

The Expressive Writing tool can be helpful in helping you change your mindset.

Mental and physical health benefits

A positive attitude towards stress significantly reduces the risk of earlier death (Keller et al., 2012). For example, the risk of dying of those who experienced a lot of stress and considered it harmful to them increased by 43% over 8 years. At the same time, the risk of dying of those who experienced a lot of stress but had a positive mindset towards stress increased by only 8%, which is less than participants who had not experienced much stress. Furthermore, a stress mindset moderates the conflict between work and home life (Hammond et al., 2021) and potentially experience better work–life balance. When anticipating high levels of workload, employees with a stress-is-enhancing mindset used more effective coping strategies at work, which allowed them to have higher levels of energy and task performance (Casper et al., 2017). Thus, the mindset can benefit your life.

Perceiving stress as debilitating is associated with poor mental and physical health (Jenkins et al., 2021). In addition, it protects against developing the symptoms of depression and anxiety (Huebschmann & Sheets, 2020). Several experimental and observational studies have demonstrated positive effects of a stress-is-enhancing mindset on physical and psychological wellbeing, on physiological, behavioural, performance, and affective outcomes in response to laboratory-induced stressors and work stress experiences (Casper et al., 2017; Crum et al., 2013, 2017; Park et al., 2018). For example, when participants had a stress-is-enhancing mindset and were challenged or threatened, their bodies produced a sharper increase of anabolic hormones responsible for growth than those who had a negative attitude towards stress (Crum et al., 2017). They also became more biased towards positive information and displayed better cognitive flexibility and higher levels of positive emotions.

Finally, stress mindset has been tested with people experiencing physical conditions. For example, a study with adults and children experiencing chronic pain showed a higher stress-is-debilitating mindset. It is suggested that the mindset is responsible for mental health outcomes and physical outcomes (Heathcote et al., 2017). However, we await more research to see whether helping patients experiencing chronic pain change their mindset impacts their perceived pain experience.

Caveat

This technique works particularly well for those with a very negative mindset about stress and has been shown to work in acute stress situations. The extent to which it will be effective in dealing with chronic stress remains to be seen.

References

Aurelius, M. (2002). *Meditations: A new translation* (G. Hays, Trans.). Modern Library.

Burke, J. (2018). Turning stress into positive energy: An evaluation of a workplace intervention. *IPPA Positive Work and Organisation: Research and Practice*, 4. Retrieved from http://www.ippanetwork.org/wp-content/uploads/2018/03/WOD-Newsletter-Issue-4-v6.pdf

Casper, A., Sonnentag, S., & Tremmel, S. (2017). Mindset matters: The role of employees' stress mindset for day-specific reactions to workload anticipation. *European Journal of Work and Organizational Psychology*, *26*(6), 798–810. doi:10.1080/1359432X.2017.1374947

Crum, A. (2022). *Stanford mind and body lab*. Retrieved from https://mbl.stanford.edu/

Crum, A. J., Corbin, W. R., Brownell, K. D., & Salovey, P. (2011). Mind over milkshakes: Mindsets, not just nutrients, determine ghrelin response. *Health Psychology*, *30*(4), 424–429.

Crum, A. J., Akinola, M., Martin, A., & Fath, S. (2017). The role of stress mindset in shaping cognitive, emotional, and physiological responses to challenging and threatening stress. *Anxiety, Stress, & Coping*, *30*(4), 379–395. doi:10.1080/10615806.2016.1275585

Crum, A. J., Salovey, P., & Achor, S. (2013). Rethinking stress: The role of mindsets in determining the stress response. *Journal of Personality and Social Psychology*, *104*(4), 716–733. doi:10.1037/a0031201

Dweck, C. S. (2017). *Mindset: Changing the way you think to fulfil your potential*. Robinson.

Frankl, V. E. (1959). *Man's search for meaning*. Washington Square Press.

Hammond, M. M., Murphy, C., & Demsky, C. A. (2021). Stress mindset and the work-family interface. *International Journal of Manpower*, *42*(1), 150–166.

Heathcote, L., Hernandez, J., Kronman, C., Mahmud, F., Crum, A., & Simons, L. (2018). (223) – 'Stress helps me learn and grow': Does stress mindset matter for children and young adults with chronic pain? *Journal of Pain*, *19*, S56. https://doi-org.elib.tcd.ie/10.1016/j.jpain.2017.12.137

Huebschmann, N. A., & Sheets, E. S. (2020). The right mindset: Stress mindset moderates the association between perceived stress and depressive symptoms. *Anxiety, Stress & Coping: An International Journal*, *33*(3), 248–255. https://doi-org.elib.tcd.ie/10.1080/10615806.2020.1736900

Jenkins, A., Weeks, M. S., & Hard, B. M. (2021). General and specific stress mindsets: Links with college student health and academic performance. *PLoS One*, *16*(9), 1–25. https://doi-org.elib.tcd.ie/10.1371/journal.pone.0256351

Keech, J. J., Hagger, M. S., & Hamilton, K. (2021). Changing stress mindsets with a novel imagery intervention: A randomized controlled trial. *Emotion*, *21*(1), 123–136. https://doi-org.elib.tcd.ie/10.1037/emo0000678.supp (Supplemental)

Keller, A., Litzelman, K., Wisk, L. E., Maddox, T., Cheng, E. R., Creswell, P. D., & Witt, W. P. (2012). Does the perception that stress affects health matter? The association with health and mortality. *Health Psychology: Official Journal of the Division of Health Psychology, American Psychological Association*, *31*(5), 677–684. https://doi.org/10.1037/a0026743

Maarsingh, B. M., Bos, J., Van Tuijn, C. F. J., & Renard, S. B. (2019). Changing stress mindset through stressjam: A virtual reality game using biofeedback. *Games for Health*, *8*(5), 326–331. https://doi-org.elib.tcd.ie/10.1089/g4h.2018.0145

O'Hare, A., & Burke, J. (Forthcoming). *Saying "yes" to stress: Examining the differences in individuals' stress levels, wellbeing and coping strategies across three levels of stress mindset.*

Pagnini, F., Cavalera, C., Volpato, E., et al. (2019). Ageing as a mindset: A study protocol to rejuvenate older adults with a counter clockwise psychological intervention. *BMJ Open, 9*, e030411. doi:10.1136/ bmjopen-2019-030411

Park, D., Yu, A., Metz, S. E., Tsukayama, E., Crum, A. J., & Duckworth, A. L. (2018). Beliefs about stress attenuate the relation among adverse life events, perceived distress, and self-control. *Child Development, 89*(6), 2059–2069. https://doi.org/10.1111/cdev.12946

Price, D. D., Finniss, D. G., & Benedetti, F. (2008). A comprehensive review of the placebo effect: Recent advances and current thought. *Annual Review of Psychology, 59*, 565–590.

Schneiderman, N., Ironson, G., & Siegel, S. D. (2005). Stress and health: Psychological, behavioral, and biological determinants. *Annual Review of Clinical Psychology, 1*, 607–628. doi:10.1146/annurev.clinpsy.1 .102803.144141

Seligman, M. E. P. (1998). *Learned optimism: How to change your mind and your life.* Pocket Books.

Yaribeygi, H., Panahi, Y., Sahraei, H., Johnston, T. P., & Sahebkar, A. (2017). The impact of stress on body function: A review. *EXCLI Journal, 16*, 1057–1072. doi:10.17179/excli2017-480

Compassion

"If you want others to be happy, practice compassion. If you want to be happy, practice compassion". Dalai Lama XIX

We have evolved as a species to differentiate between self and others; we have developed the capacity to imagine the emotional states of others, including happiness and distress. We call this empathy. Empathy can be helpful and good but sometimes overwhelming. The distinction between self and others becomes blurred during stressful times, leading to personal anxiety and distress. On the other hand, compassion can offer a solution to overwhelming empathy that causes distress. Feelings of warmth and concern characterise compassion and care for the other and strong motivation to improve the other's wellbeing. Compassion is **feeling for** and **not feeling with** the other (Singer & Klimecki, 2014).

Characteristics of empathy:

- Self-related emotion
- Negative feelings such as stress
- Poor health and burnout
- Withdrawal and non-social behaviour

Characteristics of compassion:

- Other-related emotion
- Positive emotions such as love
- Good health
- Approach and prosocial motivation

The critical point here is that compassion is about feeling for and not feeling with another human who is suffering. It is usually associated with action to offer assistance and help, however small. Compassion can extend towards others or self. In this section, we will consider tools for both.

Research-based tools

Tool 50: Loving-kindness meditation

This is an age-old Buddhist meditation practice that can help individuals cultivate compassion for themselves and others (Boellinghaus et al., 2014) and positive emotions (Zeng et al., 2015). You can use it to dampen down the self-critic that many endure. It can also be instrumental in helping us tolerate complex individuals, such as a problematic co-worker. You will find many guided versions of this practice online. However, you can also use the description that follows to practice by yourself:

- Picture yourself as you sit on a stage, looking down upon three groups of individuals.
- To your left are those you love dearly.
- In the middle are acquaintances, those you neither love nor dislike; for example, your local newsagent or bus driver.
- On the right are those whom you dislike.
- Begin with the group on the left, smile in your mind's eye, and observe them smile back at you. Try to feel the intense emotion you have for these people. Think, "I wish them health and happiness." Rest here for a moment and feel this positive emotion.
- Apply the same actions to each group as you move across to those you dislike.
- Finally, imagine your face in as much detail as possible. Wish yourself health and happiness. Try to conjure up the same positive feeling for yourself. Interestingly, many people have the most difficulty with this part of meditation. Whether you feel like it or not, act as if you love yourself and wish yourself health and happiness.

Tool 51: Volunteer (adapted from Ballard et al., 2021; Musick & Wilson, 2003)

Volunteering might have a positive impact on wellbeing; however, direct causal effects have not been confirmed. Regardless, there is enough subjective and objective evidence to show that volunteering can develop compassion and is worth engaging in. Search for an opportunity to volunteer in your community. You can do it ad hoc by embracing the opportunities that come your way. Alternatively, reflect on the people who are less fortunate than you, and think of ways to offer them support.

Tool 52: Self-compassionate writing (adapted from Johnson & O'Brien, 2013)

Think about an adverse event you've experienced recently or in the last 5 years. Now, take a piece of paper and write down responses to the three instructions that follow. Please ensure you put effort in your responses. The more effort you put in, the better the results:

1. Write a list of as many ways as you can think of in which other people have gone through a similar experience to you.
2. Write a paragraph or two in which you express kindness, love, and concern towards yourself, just as you would if you were writing to a friend.
3. Describe your feelings and emotions concerning the event in a non-emotional, objective way.

Tool 53: Self-compassion for binge eating (adapted from Kelly & Carter, 2015)

Over the next 3 weeks, follow a new routine comprising two simultaneous components:

1 REGULAR EATING

Avoid junk food; eat three meals a day and three snacks. Develop a healthy eating plan and each evening, make sure you have the next day's eating plan ready. Follow your plan closely, and each day, write down any urges you have to binge eat.

2 SELF-COMPASSION

It is common for people to be self-critical when experiencing a struggle, such as binge eating. Self-blame, however, increases our anxiety and gets in the way of our motivation to eat healthily. This is why self-compassion is a more helpful tool to prevent binge eating. In addition, when we feel cared for because we care for ourselves, we are more likely to tolerate challenges associated with the distress.

During the next 3 weeks, while you are completing your daily plan, practice self-compassion as frequently as you can. You can do it through imagery, self-talk, or letter writing. The self-compassionate mindset you are trying to get into may include the following:

- Encourage yourself with kindness to engage in behaviours that will help you prevent binge eating.
- Show yourself empathy and understanding about the struggle you experience.
- If you binge eat through this process, forgive yourself for it. Or if you are beating yourself up overdoing it in the past, forgive yourself for it.

Whenever you feel like bingeing:

- Bring back an image you associate with self-compassion or practice self-compassionate self-talk that guides you away from the food.
- Talk to yourself as you would talk to a friend who struggles, with an abundance of compassionate mindset.
- Accept that you feel distressed and that you struggle.
- Commit to taking action that is most in line with self-compassion at this point.

Variations of practice

You can practice active listening. Often, when we converse with others, we are waiting for the person to finish speaking to tell our story or get our point across. Conversely, we listen closely to the other person in active listening, providing our full attention. We show our interest and understanding through reflective body language (leaning in closer, nodding our head, mimicking movement). When the person pauses, we can ask questions that confirm we understand or are interested in learning more. Active listening can have a powerful effect on the other person, making them feel fully heard.

Also, researchers who specialise in compassion have created websites that share recommended tools for compassion. They include the Compassionate Mind Foundation, created by Professor Gilbert and his team (www.compassionatemind.co.uk/), and Kristin Neff, who focuses on self-compassion (https://self-compassion.org/). Both websites provide a list of additional resources.

Check out other tools in this book

Kindness tools and Forgiveness tools may also be useful to explore.

Mental and physical health benefits

Many researchers around the world have shown that meditation-like practices designed to cultivate compassion can have a profound positive impact on behaviour, psychology, and physical wellbeing (Greeson & Chin, 2019). For example, scientists have described how expert meditators show increased activity in several brain areas associated with emotional control and empathy compared with novices (Lutz et al., 2008). Specifically, they demonstrated how novice meditators showed slight changes in specific brain areas when exposed to neutral (restaurant), distressing (woman crying), or happy (baby laughing) sounds. In contrast, expert meditators were found to have significant increases in activity in the same brain structures. In addition, meditation practice has also been shown to improve mental health (Keng et al., 2011), especially anxiety, stress, burnout (Dunne et al., 2019), cognitive control, and emotional regulation (Tang et al., 2019). Other physical benefits include improved sleep quantity and quality (Black et al., 2015; Shallcross et al., 2019), immune function (Black & Slavich, 2016), and cardiovascular health (Levine et al., 2017).

However, not all compassionate activities involve meditation. Self-compassion can be expressed by engaging in internal self-talk, writing down compassionate thoughts, or discussing compassion with others. Self-compassion comes with a range of benefits relating to coping with unpleasant events in people's lives (Leary et al., 2007). It acts as a buffer against experiencing negative emotions when imagining distressing social events. This may be particularly useful for those with social anxiety who anticipate an event they are invited to. Self-compassion is helpful when we receive negative feedback, especially when our self-esteem is a little fragile. It also leads to people taking responsibility for the role they play in an adverse event so that they can learn from it in the future.

Shame is one of the most uncomfortable and useless emotions that makes us feel bad about ourselves. When we blame ourselves for something, we focus on what we did wrong. When we feel shame, we focus on what is wrong with us, which is particularly hurtful. Self-compassion allows us to forgo guilt for at least 2 weeks after expressing it towards ourselves (Johnson & O'Brien, 2013). Self-compassion is, therefore, very useful when it comes to reducing rumination (negative thoughts that play back in our head), anxiety, depression, and self-criticism and is especially effective at regulating eating behaviours (Ferrari et al., 2019). For example, self-compassion intervention successfully reduced binge eating and the overall global eating disorder and eating and weight concerns (Kelly & Carter, 2015). Thus, its usefulness extends beyond thoughts and emotions.

Concerning physical illness, self-compassion was very useful for patients with HIV (Brion et al., 2014). After diagnosis, they experienced less anxiety, stress, and shame when they practised higher levels of self-compassion. They were also more likely to disclose their HIV status and engage in healthy sex. Overall, self-compassion improved their adaptability and adjustment post-diagnosis. Other patients with chronic illnesses who benefited from self-compassion were diagnosed with cancer, rheumatoid arthritis, chronic pain, and diabetes (Hughes et al., 2021). Thus, self-compassion offers a lot of hope for helping individuals cope effectively with illness.

Caveat

Those who are actively grieving, survivors of abuse of any kind, and people with an extremely negative self-image should not engage in loving-kindness meditation without the support of a mental health professional.

Notes

1 The neurotransmitters adrenaline and noradrenaline are produced within seconds to activate the stress response. In contrast, stress hormones such as cortisol are produced within minutes to help counterbalance the impact of these neurotransmitters (the body always strives for balance).

References

Ballard, P. J., Daniel, S. S., Anderson, G., Nicolotti, L., Caballero Quinones, E., Lee, M., & Koehler, A. N. (2021). Incorporating volunteering into treatment for depression among adolescents: Developmental and clinical considerations. *Frontiers in Psychology*, 12(1581). doi:10.3389/fpsyg.2021.642910

Black, D. S., O'Reilly, G. A., Olmstead, R., Breen, E. C., & Irwin, M. R. (2015). Mindfulness meditation and improvement in sleep quality and daytime impairment among older adults with sleep disturbances: A randomized clinical trial. *JAMA Internal Medicine*, 175(4), 494–501. doi:10.1001/jamainternmed.2014.8081

Black, D. S., & Slavich, G. M. (2016). Mindfulness meditation and the immune system: A systematic review of randomized controlled trials. *Annals of the New York Academy of Sciences, 1373*(1), 13–24. doi:10.1111/nyas.12998

Boellinghaus, I., Jones, F. W., & Hutton, J. (2014). The role of mindfulness and loving-kindness meditation in cultivating self-compassion and other-focused concern in health care professionals. *Mindfulness, 5*(2), 129–138. doi:10.1007/s12671-012-0158-6

Brion, J. M., Leary, M. R., & Drabkin, A. S. (2014). Self-compassion and reactions to serious illness: The case of HIV. *Journal of Health Psychology, 19*(2), 218–229. https://doi-org.elib.tcd.ie/10.1177/1359105312467391

Dunne, P. J., Lynch, J., Prihodova, L., O'Leary, C., Ghoreyshi, A., Basdeo, S. A., . . . White, B. (2019). Burnout in the emergency department: Randomized controlled trial of an attention-based training program. *Journal of Integrative Medicine*. doi:10.1016/j.joim.2019.03.009

Ferrari, M., Hunt, C., Harrysunker, A., Abbott, M. J., Beath, A. P., & Einstein, D. A. (2019). Self-compassion interventions and psychosocial outcomes: A meta-analysis of RCTs. *Mindfulness, 10*(8), 1455–1473. https://doi-org.elib.tcd.ie/10.1007/s12671-019-01134-6

Greeson, J. M., & Chin, G. R. (2019). Mindfulness and physical disease: A concise review. *Current Opinion in Psychology, 28*, 204–210. https://doi.org/10.1016/j.copsyc.2018.12.014

Hughes, M., Brown, S. L., Campbell, S., Dandy, S., & Cherry, M. G. (2021). Self-compassion and anxiety and depression in chronic physical illness populations: A systematic review. *Mindfulness, 12*(7), 1597–1610. https://doi-org.elib.tcd.ie/10.1007/s12671-021-01602-y

Johnson, E. A., & O'Brien, K. A. (2013). Self-compassion soothes the savage ego-threat system: Effects on negative affect, shame, rumination, and depressive symptoms. *Journal of Social and Clinical Psychology, 32*(9), 939–963. https://doi-org.elib.tcd.ie/10.1521/jscp.2013.32.9.939

Kelly, A. C., & Carter, J. C. (2015). Self-compassion training for binge eating disorder: A pilot randomized controlled trial. *Psychology & Psychotherapy: Theory, Research & Practice, 88*(3), 285–303. https://doi-org.elib.tcd.ie/10.1111/papt.12044

Keng, S. L., Smoski, M. J., & Robins, C. J. (2011). Effects of mindfulness on psychological health: A review of empirical studies. *Clinical Psychology Review, 31*(6), 1041–1056. doi:10.1016/j.cpr.2011.04.006

Leary, M. R., Tate, E. B., Adams, C. E., Batts Allen, A., & Hancock, J. (2007). Self-compassion and reactions to unpleasant self-relevant events: The implications of treating oneself kindly. *Journal of Personality and Social Psychology, 92*(5), 887–904. https://doi-org.elib.tcd.ie/10.1037/0022-3514.92.5.887

Levine, G. N., Lange, R. A., Bairey-Merz, C. N., Davidson, R. J., Jamerson, K., Mehta, P. K., . . . Smith, S. C., Jr. (2017). Meditation and cardiovascular risk reduction: A scientific statement from the American heart association. *Journal of the American Heart Association, 6*(10). doi:10.1161/jaha.117.002218

Lutz, A., Brefczynski-Lewis, J., Johnstone, T., & Davidson, R. J. (2008). Regulation of the neural circuitry of emotion by compassion meditation: Effects of meditative expertise. *PLoS One, 3*(3), e1897. doi:10.1371/journal.pone.0001897

Musick, M. A., & Wilson, J. (2003). Volunteering and depression: The role of psychological and social resources in different age groups. *Social Science & Medicine*, *56*(2), 259–269. doi:10.1016/s0277-9536(02)00025-4

Shallcross, A. J., Visvanathan, P. D., Sperber, S. H., & Duberstein, Z. T. (2019). Waking up to the problem of sleep: Can mindfulness help? A review of theory and evidence for the effects of mindfulness for sleep. *Current Opinion in Psychology*, *28*, 37–41. https://doi.org/10.1016/j.copsyc.2018.10.005

Singer, T., & Klimecki, O. M. (2014). Empathy and compassion. *Current Biology*, *24*(18), R875–R878. https://doi.org/10.1016/j.cub.2014.06.054

Tang, Y.-Y., Tang, R., Rothbart, M. K., & Posner, M. I. (2019). Frontal theta activity and white matter plasticity following mindfulness meditation. *Current Opinion in Psychology*, *28*, 294–297. https://doi.org/10.1016/j.copsyc.2019.04.004

Zeng, X., Chiu, C. P. K., Wang, R., Oei, T. P. S., & Leung, F. Y. K. (2015). The effect of loving-kindness meditation on positive emotions: A meta-analytic review. *Frontiers in Psychology*, *6*. doi:10.3389/fpsyg.2015.01693

Your reflection space

Which coping tools would you like to try? Why?
Which activities did you find most useful? How did you tweak them?

5 Feeling-good tools

Feeling-good tools are all about experiencing more positive than negative emotions. For years, we have viewed positive emotions as poor cousins of negative emotions. Some of the main conceptualisations of emotions, such as Ekman's basic emotions model, comprised six emotions, five of which were negative. Researchers, therefore, examined in detail the meaning, prevalence, and benefits of negative emotions and assumed that positive emotions are merely the opposite of negative emotions. Whilst negative emotions served an essential evolutionary purpose, aiding survival, positive emotions made us happy. Until one day when an American researcher, Alice Isen, published a series of experiments demonstrating the invaluable effect of positive emotions on decision-making (Isen, 1993).

Following Isen, Barbara Fredrickson (2001) created a Broaden and Build theory that explained the role positive emotions play in our lives. The theory and its evidence show that positive emotions broaden our perspective. Thus, when experiencing challenging situations in life, we can see more creative ways to resolve them and notice opportunities. They also build our resources for the future. Those include:

- Intellectual resources, e.g. problem-solving
- Physical resources, e.g. cardiovascular health
- Social resources, e.g. maintaining relationships
- Psychological resources, e.g. optimism

Finally, another important role that positive emotions play is that they undo the effect of negative emotions. Therefore, when they follow an adverse event, we can bounce back faster and recover faster from it.

The importance of experiencing positive emotions has been long acknowledged and appreciated by therapists, who often encourage their clients to find ways to experience positive emotions. Positive emotions

DOI: 10.4324/9781003279594-7

help people get unstuck, open up their minds, and help them become more resilient. Furthermore, recognising emotions, especially their delightful variety, can help us express ourselves more effectively when describing our life experiences, ultimately improving our emotional intelligence and wellbeing (Barret, 2020). This is why becoming aware of our emotions, learning to name them, and experiencing their daily variety is of utmost importance.

One of our clients, who experienced depression, realised that their busy life resulted in experiencing more hassles than pleasures every day. This is why, as a personal experiment, he began to plan pleasurable activities while in the shower every morning. He planned for at least three things he wanted to do during the day that gave him a positive emotional boost. These included having something special for his lunch, going to the staff canteen during his morning break to chat with colleagues, going for a short walk during lunch break, aimless browsing through a social networking site, checking out videos, and listening to 10 minutes of meditation before he entered his busy home with five children trying to attract his attention. Some days, he challenged himself by aiming to experience specific positive emotions, such as planning for awe, hope, gratitude, and amusement. He noticed that on the days when he planned positive activities, he experienced more positive emotions. Soon, this simple experiment became his new habit improving his life.

This chapter provides you with various tools that will help you enhance your positive emotions and help you feel good. However, these tools are not exclusive, as most of the tools in this book boost some of our positive emotions.

Feeling-good tools include:

1 Reminiscing
2 Strengths
3 Gratitude
4 Music
5 Visiting an art gallery

References

Barrett, L. F. (2020). *How emotions are made*. Pan Macmillan.
Fredrickson, B. L. (2001). The role of positive emotions in positive psychology: The broaden-and-build theory of positive emotions. *American Psychologist*, *56*(3), 218–226. https://doi-org.elib.tcd.ie/10.1037/0003-066X.56.3.218
Isen, A. M. (1993). Positive affect and decision making. In M. Lewis & J. M. Haviland (Eds.), *Handbook of emotions* (pp. 261–277). The Guilford Press.

Reminiscing

Human beings have a magical power to travel across all time perspectives, past, present, and future. This section will discuss the beneficial effect of using our past experiences to enhance our wellbeing today and tomorrow. This is what we naturally do when we get older, by telling stories about the good old days, but we can just as well use this tool to boost our wellbeing at any time of our lives and in all circumstances. Reminiscence is a process by which we think, write or tell others about our past experiences that we find meaningful (Pinquart & Forstmeier, 2012). Reminiscence comes in two forms. Firstly, we can reminisce about ad hoc events from the past that gave us a positive boost, which we can re-experience in the present. Secondly, we can tell our life stories. Describing our lives is a complex process that includes incorporating positive and negative events and their interaction with each other and subsequent life evaluation that follows, whereas reminiscing about ad hoc positive events comprises simple reminiscence, which is what this section is about.

Research-based tools

Tool 54: Reminiscence (adapted from Bryant et al., 2004)

Write down a list of several positive memories from the past. Then, set aside 10 min to sit quietly once or twice a day over the next week. Select one memory at a time to reflect on. You can do it by sitting down, taking a few deep breaths in and out, closing your eyes, and thinking intensely about the memory. You will see images emerging with this memory, followed by emotions. Allow your mind to wander while you bask in the positive events from your past.

Tool 55: Intensely positive experiences (adapted from Burton & King, 2004)

Consider some of the happiest moments in your life, moments that have given you an ecstatic feeling. This could include falling in love, your baby being born, being moved by music, or another memorable time of your life. Select one memory, and over the next 15 to 20 minutes, write about it in as much detail as you can. Don't worry about any mistakes, spelling, or grammar. Instead, focus on your thoughts, feelings, emotions, circumstances, people around you, etc. Then, try to re-experience the positive emotions this happy moment gave you.

Variations of practice

Wing and colleagues (2006) varied the intensely positive experience tool by asking participants to reflect on how, in the future, they could tap into the positive emotions that they had experienced in the past, so you may try to do it too. Some researchers (e.g. Habermas & Paha, 2000) recommended that to aid reminiscence, you can use souvenirs or memorabilia or review your old photographs, which will bring back the good memories. Also, instead of writing, you may choose to daydream about the past or chat with a friend about the good old days, which may evoke the same burst of positive emotions.

Mental and physical health benefits

Positive reminiscence is a hallmark of happiness and predicts the experience of high levels of positive emotions (Parks et al., 2013). A 6-week programme that focused on helping clients reminiscent of the past not only enhanced their wellbeing but also reduced the symptoms of depression and anxiety (Zauszniewski et al., 2004). It is as if the good memories took over the headspace occupied by bad memories. A meta-analysis of reminiscing interventions across 128 studies showed that they improved psychological wellbeing, cognitive performance, and symptoms of depression and chronic physical disease, with most of the changes maintained at follow-up a week, month or several months later (Pinquart & Forstmeier, 2012). In addition to the mental health benefits, practising the Intense Positive Experience tool for 20 minutes over 3 days improved participants' moods, but more importantly, it also improved their physical health to an extent whereby 3 months later, they reported fewer visits to the doctor than the control group (Burton & King, 2004). Thus, reminiscence has a positive impact on both our mental and physical health.

Furthermore, reminiscence therapy, which is a strength-based approach drawing from preserved positive memories has been used extensively with people diagnosed with various forms of dementia (Macleod et al., 2021). Apart from giving patients a boost of positive emotions, it helped them create life meaning and build a sense of identity of the limited memories they have left. For example, a 5-week intense therapy with Alzheimer's patients significantly improved their autobiographic memory, thus showing an improvement in their cognitive skills despite considerable decline (Kirk et al., 2018). Reminiscence intervention has also been offered via telephone to patients diagnosed with cancer while undergoing post-operative chemotherapy, and it resulted in a significant reduction of their symptoms of depression (Dong et al., 2018). Thus, reminiscence is useful for prompting positive wellbeing outcomes as well as reducing cognitive decline.

Caveat

While reminiscing about the good old days is useful, briefly thinking about some of the negative situations from the past may help you balance your emotions and ensure you can learn from your mistakes (Zimbardo & Boyd, 1999).

References

Bryant, F. B., Smart, C. M., & King, S. P. (2004). *(PDF) using the past to enhance the present: Boosting happiness through positive reminiscence.* Retrieved December 17, 2021, from www.researchgate.net/publication/23545544_Using_the_Past_to_Enhance_the_Present_Boosting_Happiness_Through_Positive_Reminiscence

Burton, C. M., & King, L. A. (2004). The health benefits of writing about intensely positive experiences. *Journal of Research in Personality, 38*(2), 150–163. https://doi-org.elib.tcd.ie/10.1016/S0092-6566(03)00058-8

Dong, J., Gruda, N., Lam, S. K., Li, X., & Duan, Z. (2018). Effects of elevated CO_2 on nutritional quality of vegetables: A review. *Frontiers in Plant Science, 9*, 924. https://doi-org.elib.tcd.ie/10.3389/fpls.2018.00924

Habermas, T., & Paha, C. (2000). Souvenirs and other personal objects: Reminding of past events and significant others in the transition to university. In J. D. Webster & B. K. Haight (Eds.), *Critical advances in reminiscence work: From theory to application* (pp. 123–139). Springer.

Kirk, M., Rasmussen, K. W., Overgaard, S. B., & Berntsen, D. (2019). Five weeks of immersive reminiscence therapy improves autobiographical memory in Alzheimer's disease. *Memory, 27*(4), 441–454. https://doi-org.elib.tcd.ie/10.1080/09658211.2018.1515960

Macleod, F., Storey, L., Rushe, T., & McLaughlin, K. (2021). Towards an increased understanding of reminiscence therapy for people with dementia: A narrative analysis. *Dementia* (14713012), *20*(4), 1375–1407. https://doi-org.elib.tcd.ie/10.1177/1471301220941275

Parks, A. C., Schueller, S. M., & Tasimi, A. (2013). Increasing happiness in the general population: Empirically supported self-help? In S. A. David, I. Boniwell, & A. C. Ayers (Eds.), *The Oxford handbook of happiness* (pp. 962–977). Oxford University Press.

Pinquart, M., & Forstmeier, S. (2012). Effects of reminiscence interventions on psychosocial outcomes: A meta-analysis. *Aging & Mental Health, 16*(5), 541–558. https://doi-org.elib.tcd.ie/10.1080/13607863.2011.651434

Wing, J. F., Schutte, N. S., & Byrne, B. (2006). The effect of positive writing on emotional intelligence and life satisfaction. *Journal of Clinical Psychology, 62*(10), 1291–1302. https://doi-org.elib.tcd.ie/10.1002/jclp.20292

Zauszniewski, J. A., Eggenschwiler, K., Preechawong, S., Chung, W., Airey, T. F., . . . Roberts, B. L. (2004). Focused reflection reminiscence group for elders: Implementation and evaluation. *Journal of Applied Gerontology, 23*, 429–442.

Zimbardo, P. G., & Boyd, J. N. (1999). Putting time in perspective: A valid, reliable individual-differences metric. *Journal of Personality and Social Psychology, 77*(6), 1271–1288. https://doi.org/10.1037/0022-3514.77.6.1271

Strengths

Human beings are much more attuned to the negative than the positive – we are more affected by bad events than by good and pay more attention to and remember negative information more thoroughly than good (Baumeister et al., 2001). We are generally more aware of our vulnerabilities and frailties than our strengths. One of the significant contributions of positive psychology has been its focus on identifying and using our character strengths. Not only does this allow us to build and utilise our strengths, but it also helps balance our negative biases.

Character strengths are defined as positive capacities and traits that are valued, do not diminish others, and which we find personally fulfilling (Peterson & Seligman, 2004). Character strengths are our positive capacities for thinking, feeling, and behaving and are core components of our psychological identity.

Over the past 20 or so years, researchers have developed several validated methods for measuring our strengths and optimising their use. These include the Clifton Strengths Finder (www.strengthsfinder), the Strengths Profile (www.strengthsprofile.com), and the VIA Character Strengths Questionnaire (www.viacharacter.org). Here, we will focus on the VIA system. The VIA classification of strengths and virtues, available free at www.viacharacter.org, allows you to rate yourself on 24 character strengths organised into six virtues. Completing the VIA questionnaire provides a rank order of your 24 strengths and allows you to develop and use them more effectively.

The six virtues and 24 character strengths measured by the VIA questionnaire

Virtue	Associated Character Strengths
Wisdom	Creativity, Curiosity, Judgement, Love of Learning, Perspective
Courage	Bravery, Perseverance, Honesty, Zest
Humanity	Love, Kindness, Social Intelligence
Justice	Teamwork, Fairness, Leadership
Temperance	Forgiveness, Humility, Prudence, Self-Regulation
Transcendence	Appreciation of Beauty and Excellence, Gratitude, Hope, Humour, Spirituality

Source: www.viacharacter.org

Research-based tools

Tool 56: Strength assessment (Niemiec & McGrath, 2019)

The first step is to complete the VIA character strength assessment (www.viacharacter.org), examine your feedback, and become aware of all 24 strengths and how they relate to you. We often take our strengths for granted, and the important point here is to become more aware of and use your strengths in your daily life in a more mindful way. Not only does this make you more effective in using your strengths, it also acts as a counterweight to the negativity we discussed at the start of this section. As you become more aware of your own strengths and how you can use them, try also to spot signature strengths in others.

Tool 57: Use your signature strengths (adapted from Seligman et al., 2005)

1. Complete the VIA character strengths assessment (www.viacharacter.org)
2. While all 24 strengths are of interest, focus on your top five to seven strengths, your *signature strengths*.
3. Every day for the next week, use your top (signature) strengths in a new and different way. For example, you might use Love of Learning to find new ways to overcome challenges; the strength of Kindness to do a favour for a friend; the strength of Zest to do something because you really want to do it, not because you think you should.

Tool 58: Use your lesser strengths (adapted from Proyer et al., 2015)

1. Complete the VIA character strengths assessment (www.viacharacter.org).
2. Select your lesser strengths (at the bottom of your report), and every day over the next week, try to use them in a new and different way. If you find yourself in a new environment or are interacting with a new person, using your strengths in this novel situation may be considered new and different. You can apply your strengths in whatever way you wish. It is up to you.

Tool 59: Job as a calling (adapted from Harzer & Ruch, 2016)

Broadly speaking, you can have three attitudes towards work: you can perceive your job as a:

- calling (you do it for the sake of it, you have intrinsic motivation to do it)
- career (you are motivated by progressing your career), or
- just a job, a source of income for you.

Perceiving your job as a calling is associated with a range of psychological benefits. To help you experience them, please follow this four-step process:

1. Complete your VIA character assessment (www.viacharacter.org).
2. Think about your daily activities and tasks at work.
3. Consider how you currently use your strengths.
4. Develop an if–then plan on how you can use your character strengths more often at work. An if–then plan works like this: If I am asked to do extra work, then I will use my strength of Courage and say "not now".
5. Character strengths can help you turn your job from just a job to a calling. Select your five top (signature) strengths and come up with ways in which you can use them daily at work.

Tool 60: Strengths – family contract (adapted from Waters, 2020)

1. Gather all members of your family together and discuss what makes your family happy.
2. Now, set up two family goals for enhancing your happiness using your earlier discussion.
3. Discuss how each of your family members can use their individual strengths to help the family meet your happiness goals.
4. Every day over the next week, spot strengths in your family members, and tell them when you see them use their strengths.
5. Meet at the end of the week to discuss how well you progressed your family goals.
6. If you wish to continue with this activity, repeat steps 3 to 5 weekly.

Variations in practice

Think of new ways you can use your strengths to accomplish your goals, e.g. improve your relationships, move you towards your goals, and overcome difficulties. One particularly interesting approach to identifying strengths and learning about them is provided by Niemiec and Wedding

(2014) in their book *Positive Psychology at the Movies*. The authors systematically discussed each of the 24 signature strengths in depth and suggested movies to help understand the strengths in more depth. Here are a few films related to some of the strengths to get you started: Bravery: *Hotel Rwanda*; Creativity: *Life Is Beautiful*; Fairness: *12 Angry Men*; Humour: *Zorba the Greek*; Kindness: *Amélie*.

Mental and physical health benefits

We can improve and develop our character strengths, and when we express them, we feel happier, more connected, and more productive (Niemiec & McGrath, 2019). A systematic review of strengths interventions found that they have a significant impact on enhancing life satisfaction (Schutte & Malouff, 2019). Furthermore, using strengths at work results in higher levels of employee engagement (Bakker & Wingerden, 2021) and psychological flourishing (Hone et al., 2015).

There is also good evidence that identifying and using our strengths contribute to happiness, wellbeing, and physical health not only in healthy people but also in patients with chronic conditions, such as traumatic brain injury, breast cancer, schizoaffective disorder, psychosis, depression, and anxiety disorder (Yan et al., 2020). Using character strengths results in increase of happiness, hope, self-esteem, resilience, quality of life, and life satisfaction, to mention but a few outcomes. Furthermore, increasingly, strengths have been used with individuals with addiction (Selvam, 2015). Thus, character strengths are a useful tool for both clinical and non-clinical populations.

Caveat

We can underuse or overuse any of our character strengths, and when this happens, we no longer get the benefits of them. For example, overusing curiosity can lead to nosiness, underusing it to disinterest. Overusing kindness can lead to intrusiveness, underusing it to indifference. Over- or underuse becomes a problem when it negatively affects ourselves and others. According to Niemiec (2018), the best way to avoid this is to think of each strength as a continuum in terms of how you express it in a given situation or context, where the centre is a balanced, optimal use in terms of the right amount for the situation. Becoming more aware of how we might be over- or underusing our strengths and how this might be affecting others can make us more mindful and more positive and also provide us with a stimulus for reflection and development.

References

Bakker, A. B., & van Wingerden, J. (2021). Do personal resources and strengths use increase work engagement? The effects of a training intervention. *Journal of Occupational Health Psychology*, *26*(1), 20–30. https://doi-org.elib.tcd.ie/10.1037/ocp0000266

Baumeister, R. F., Bratslavsky, E., Finkenaeuer, C., & Vohs, K. D. (2001). Bad is stronger than good. *Review of General Psychology*, *5*(4), 323–370.

Harzer, C., & Ruch, W. (2016). Your strengths are calling: Preliminary results of a web-based strengths intervention to increase calling. *Journal of Happiness Studies*, *17*(6), 2237–2256. https://doi-org.elib.tcd.ie/10.1007/s10902-015-9692-y

Hone, L. C., Jarden, A., Duncan, S., & Schofield, G. M. (2015). Flourishing in New Zealand workers: Associations with lifestyle behaviors, physical health, psychosocial, and work-related indicators. *Journal of Occupational and Environmental Medicine*, *57*(9), 973–983. https://doi.org/10.1097/JOM.0000000000000508

Niemiec, R. M. (2018). *Character strengths interventions: A field-guide for practitioners*. Hogrefe.

Niemiec, R. M., & McGrath, R. E. (2019). *The power of character strengths: Appreciate and ignite your positive personality*. The VIA Institute on Character.

Niemiec, R. M., & Wedding, D. (2014). *Positive psychology at the movies: Using films to build character strengths and well-being* (2nd ed.). Hogrefe.

Peterson, C., & Seligman, M. E. P. (2004). *Character strengths and virtues: A handbook and classification*. American Psychological Association; Oxford University Press.

Proyer, R. T., Gander, F., Wellenzohn, S., & Ruch, W. (2015). Strengths-based positive psychology interventions: A randomized placebo-controlled online trial on long-term effects for a signature strengths- vs a lesser strengths-intervention. *Frontiers in Psychology*, *6*. https://doi-org.elib.tcd.ie/10.3389/fpsyg.2015.00456

Schutte, N. S., & Malouff, J. M. (2019). The impact of signature character strengths interventions: A meta-analysis. *Journal of Happiness Studies*, *20*(4), 1179–1196. https://doi-org.elib.tcd.ie/10.1007/s10902-018-9990-2

Seligman, M. E. P., Steen, T. A., Park, N., & Peterson, C. (2005). Positive psychology progress: Empirical validation of interventions. *American Psychologist*, *60*(5), 410–421.

Selvam, S. G. (2015). Positive psychology's character strengths in addiction-spirituality research: A qualitative systematic literature review. *Qualitative Report*, *20*(4), 376–405.

Waters, L. (2020). Using positive psychology interventions to strengthen family happiness: A family systems approach. *Journal of Positive Psychology*, *15*(5), 645–652. https://doi-org.elib.tcd.ie/10.1080/17439760.2020.1789704

Yan, T., Chan, C. W. H., Chow, K. M., Zheng, W., & Sun, M. (2020). A systematic review of character strengths-based intervention on psychological wellbeing of patients suffering from chronic illness. *Journal of Advanced Nursing, 76*(7), 1567–1580.

Gratitude

Gratitude is an expression of thankfulness for whom or what we have in our lives. It is a skill we develop as we grow, which does not come naturally. This is why children need to be reminded to thank others for their kindness, e.g. say "thank you" after receiving a gift. Equally, adults need to become aware of what they are grateful for and reflect on it regularly, e.g. being thankful for the friends in your life. The practice of gratitude usually starts by reflecting on important things we are grateful for, such as our home and people in our lives. The more we do it, the more we can notice the small things in our lives for which we are thankful, e.g. that old lady smiling at us briefly on the train or 10 minutes of respite when the kids are preoccupied with their new toy. Gratitude is also one of the most researched tools in psychology, with strong evidence for enhancing wellbeing.

Research-based tools

Tool 61: Five good things (adapted from Emmons & McCullough, 2003)

Write down five things for which you are thankful or grateful. Then, consider the events from the past week, both big and small, to help you do it.

Tool 62: Gratitude at work (adapted from Waters, 2015)

Over the next 2 weeks, write a gratitude diary that will allow you to reflect on what you are grateful for after work. Then, after 2 weeks, write an email to a colleague in which you thank them for the support they gave in the last 2 weeks.

Tool 63: Gratitude list with a twist (Seligman, 2011)

Every night before going to bed, set aside 10 minutes to write down three things that went well for you today and reflect on why they happened. In the original activity, the researchers asked people to do this activity for a week, but you may decide on what duration best suits you and your lifestyle.

Tool 64: Gratitude letter and/or visit (Stone et al., 2021)

Take a moment to think back over the past several years of your life and remember an instance when someone did something for you for which you are extremely grateful. For example, think of the people – parents, relatives, friends, teachers, coaches, teammates, employers, and so on – who have been especially kind to you but have never heard you express your gratitude. For the next 15 minutes, write a letter to one of these individuals. Use the instructions that follow to help guide you through this process:

1. Use whatever letter format you like but remember to write as though you directly address the individual. If it is helpful to head the letter "Dear so-and-so", or end with

    "Sincerely, XXX", feel free to do so.
2. Do not worry about perfect grammar and spelling.
3. Describe in specific terms why you are grateful to this individual and how the individual's behaviour affected your life.
4. Describe what you are doing now and how you often remember their efforts.

You may also deliver the letter by post or in person as a variation of this activity.

Variations of practice

You don't need to express gratitude or become a benefactor of gratitude to experience its benefits. The latest research is showing that witnessing gratitude makes us more grateful (Algoe et al., 2020). Therefore, to boost the experience of this emotion, you may try to spend time in places where people express gratitude or watch movies, online clips, or news in which people thank each other frequently.

Some of us use a gratitude jar or gratitude board where we post notes of gratitude throughout the week and then reflect on them over the weekend. We can also procure a "gratitude partner" to share our appreciation. For example, some researchers asked people to reflect on "three things I'm lucky for", enhancing wellbeing (Shankland & Rosset, 2017).

In addition, the WWW activity (want went well) is a helpful way to start a meeting in the workplace. Finally, gratitude supported by coaching after completing a gratitude activity is reported to accelerate the experience of meaning in life; thus, you could use coaching in tandem with practising gratitude for better results (Trom & Burke, 2021).

Mental and physical health benefits

Gratitude interventions are effective in reducing mood disorders, such as depression and anxiety (Cregg & Cheavens, 2021), as well as suicide ideation (Lin, 2021). They are also used as quality-of-life interventions in patients with multiple sclerosis (Crouch et al., 2020), cancer (Sztachańska et al., 2019), neuromuscular disease (Emmons & McCullough, 2003), and in palliative care (Althaus et al., 2018).

In relation to physiological health, practising gratitude is associated with improved sleep (Boggiss et al., 2020), regulating heart rate, and helping individuals cope with stressful events more effectively (Redwine et al., 2016). Compared with other psychological tools, gratitude activities increased individuals' wellbeing the most (Davis et al., 2016).

Caveats

Overusing gratitude may cause boredom. When it is used every day for 2 or more weeks, it may become a chore. This is why, it is useful to start off by engaging with it daily. As soon as you start becoming bored with it, reduce the frequency to once or twice a week, or choose to do it on an ad hoc basis. That said, some individuals have a predisposition (strength) to gratitude and love this activity so much that they want to do it regularly for years without feeling bored with it. The best thing is to do what works for you. Furthermore, please note that there are cultural differences in the effect of gratitude tools applied in collectivist and individualist cultures (Shin et al., 2020). However, further research is needed to identify the intricacies of these differences.

References

Algoe, S. B., Dwyer, P. C., Younge, A., & Oveis, C. (2020). A new perspective on the social functions of emotions: Gratitude and the witnessing effect. *Journal of Personality and Social Psychology, 119*(1), 40–74. https://doi.org/10.1037/pspi0000202

Althaus, B., Borasio, G. D., & Bernard, M. (2018). Gratitude at the end of life: A promising lead for palliative care. *Journal of Palliative Medicine, 21*(11), 1566–1572. doi:10.1089/jpm.2018.0027

Boggiss, A. L., Consedine, N. S., Brenton-Peters, J. M., Hofman, P. L., & Serlachius, A. S. (2020). A systematic review of gratitude interventions: Effects on physical health and health behaviors. *Journal of Psychosomatic Research, 135*. https://doi-org. elib.tcd.ie/10.1016/j.jpsychores.2020.110165

Cregg, D. R., & Cheavens, J. S. (2021). Gratitude interventions: Effective self-help? A meta-analysis of the impact on symptoms of depression and anxiety. *Journal of Happiness Studies, 22*(1), 413–445. doi:10.1007/s10902-020-00236-6

Crouch, T. A., Verdi, E. K., & Erickson, T. M. (2020). Gratitude is positively associated with quality of life in multiple sclerosis. *Rehabilitation Psychology, 65*(3), 231–238. doi:10.1037/rep0000319

Davis, D. E., Choe, E., Meyers, J., Varjas, K., Gifford, A., Quinn, A., Van Tongeren, D. R., Wade, N., Hook, J. N., Griffin, B. J., & Worthington Jr., E. L. (2016). Thankful for the little things: A meta-analysis of gratitude interventions. *Journal of Counseling Psychology, 63*(1), 20–31. https://doi-org.elib.tcd.ie/10.1037/cou0000107

Emmons, R. A., & McCullough, M. E. (2003). Counting blessings versus burdens: An experimental investigation of gratitude and subjective wellbeing in daily life. *Journal of Personality and Social Psychology, 84*(2), 377–389. doi:10.1037/0022-3514.84.2.377

Lin, C.-C. (2021). The effects of gratitude on suicidal ideation among late adolescence: A mediational chain. *Current Psychology, 40*(5), 2242–2250. doi:10.1007/s12144-019-0159-x

Redwine, L. S., Henry, B. L., Pung, M. A., Wilson, K., Chinh, K., Knight, B., . . . Mills, P. J. (2016). Pilot randomized study of a gratitude journaling intervention on heart rate variability and inflammatory biomarkers in patients with stage B heart failure. *Psychosomatic Medicine, 78*(6), 667–676. doi:10.1097/PSY.0000000000000316

Seligman, M. E. P. (2011). *Flourish: A visionary new understanding of happiness and wellbeing*. Atria.

Shankland, R., & Rosset, E. (2017). Review of brief school-based positive psychological interventions: A taster for teachers and educators. *Educational Psychology Review, 29*(2), 363–392. doi:10.1007/s10648-016-9357-3

Shin, L. J., Armenta, C. N., Kamble, S. V., Chang, S.-L., Wu, H.-Y., & Lyubomirsky, S. (2020). Gratitude in collectivist and individualist cultures. *The Journal of Positive Psychology*. doi:10.1080/17439760.2020.1789699

Stone, B. M., Lindt, J. D., Rabinovich, N. E., & Gilbert, D. G. (2021). Effects of the gratitude letter and positive attention bias modification on attentional deployment and emotional states. *Journal of Happiness Studies: An Interdisciplinary Forum on Subjective Well-Being*. https://doi.org/10.1007/s10902-021-00377-2

Sztachańska, J., Krejtz, I., & Nezlek, J. B. (2019). Using a gratitude intervention to improve the lives of women with breast cancer: A daily diary study. *Frontiers in Psychology, 10*. doi:10.3389/fpsyg.2019.01365

Trom, P., & Burke, J. (2021). Positive psychology intervention (ppi) coaching: An experimental application of coaching to improve the effectiveness of a gratitude intervention. *Coaching: An International Journal of Theory, Research and Practice*. doi:10.1080/17521882.2021.1936585

Waters, L., & Stokes, H. (2015). Positive education for school leaders: Exploring the effects of emotion-gratitude and action-gratitude. *Australian Educational and Developmental Psychologist, 32*(1), 1–22.

Music

Ludwig van Beethoven famously said that "music can change the world". However, it can also change something much more important: the people who live in this world. Music therapy has been long renowned for its positive effect in helping non-verbal children with autism connect in ways they have not connected before (Sharda et al., 2018), in aiding adults with depression to find a new lease on life (Chan et al., 2009), or helping us all to find more joy in our daily existence. Whether we like it or not, all music we listen to changes our emotional state, with some tunes inducing happiness while other tunes prompting sadness, which is received not only at a conscious level but also as a result of unconscious physiological reactions that ultimately affect our psyche (Ribeiro et al., 2019). When used wisely, music can help us enhance our wellbeing instead of dampening our mood. Experiencing higher levels of positive emotions and uplifting moods will affect what we do with our lives. Thus, Beethoven may have been correct to say that music can change the world, but he forgot to mention that it does it one person at a time. As such, music as an activity can be roughly divided into the practices of making music and listening to it. There is a large field of music therapy. In this section, we talk about the benefits of music as a daily activity, not a treatment supported by a professional.

Research-based tools

Tool 65: Listening to uplifting music of your choice (adapted from Sergeant & Mongrain, 2011).

Create your intervention playlist and listen to 3-4 uplifting songs of your choosing each day for 7 days. You may continue practising this exercise for as long as you wish if it works for you.

Tool 66: Music before sleep (adapted from Chan et al., 2009)

Listen to music of your choice for 30 minutes a day for a month; ideally, shortly before going to bed. The type of music recommended in this experiment had a tempo of 60 to 80 beats a minute without accented beats, percussive characteristics, or syncopation. For example, Western classical (e.g. Beethoven's Symphony No. 5), Western jazz (e.g. "April in Paris", "Dreamsville"), Chinese classical (e.g. "TAO", "Lord of Wind"), and Asian classical (e.g. "Everlasting Road"). However, you may choose to listen to any music that has the same feel-good effect on you.

Tool 67: Make music (adapted from Conner et al., 2018)

Engage in a creative musical activity daily (make music, write a song, learn to play an instrument, sing). Don't judge yourself, and don't worry if you are not good at it. Just have fun being imperfect.

Variations of practice

When working with clients, we often recommend that they create their own positive music playlist and play it whenever they need to lift their mood (e.g. after a bad day, an argument with their spouse, or when they wake up on the wrong side of the bed). Our automatic reaction is to listen to tunes that reflect our mood. For example, when we experience disappointment in love, we are drawn towards sad music; when we are angry, we might want to listen to music that reflects our emotion. But the trick is to manage our emotions by changing the tune we listen to – when feeling sad, forcing ourselves to listen to more upbeat and hopeful music, and when feeling angry, selecting calmer tunes to relax us. Choosing to listen to music that brings a more uplifting mood can help us enhance our wellbeing. Also, we suggested that our clients, when feeling low, put on the radio. Many of them mentioned how this simple activity raised their mood and helped them experience more positive emotions, and in the case of radio discussions with some music intertwined, it allowed them to temporarily distract themselves from their own thoughts and focus on more existential ideas. Some also added that as they turned the radio on and stumbled upon a tune they had not heard for a long time, they found themselves dancing in the kitchen to the sound of music, making themselves feel even happier. While, to our knowledge, we don't have experimental studies to confirm the effectiveness of these simple techniques for enhancing our mood, we recommend you try it anyway. If it works for some of our clients, it could work for you.

Chanting prayer and yoga mantras have been studied for their rhythmic formulas (Bernardi et al., 2001). The rhythms are usually recited six times a minute. This type of rhythmic chanting functions to slow breathing, increasing heart rate variability and baroreflex sensitivity, both implicated in heart health. The instructions for such practice are: recite the "typical yoga mantra 'om mani padme om' . . . with an 'alive' resonance voice . . . listen to the sound produced and let it flow freely and then complete the expiration comfortably after the end of the mantra" (Bernardi et al., 2001, p. 23).

Mental and physical health benefits

In a recent review of the benefits of music practice and participation, Croom (2015) argues that music impacts all aspects of wellbeing, i.e. positive emotion, engagement, relationships, meaning, and achievement (PERMA: Seligman, 2011). Music has been shown to have multiple benefits that contribute to wellbeing, including increased positive emotion and the experience of flow or deep engagement. Listening to music together has been argued to create peer cohesion and social relatedness, thus contributing to positive relationships. Literature on the role of music and our identity shows that music also supports the wellbeing factor of meaning (Croom, 2015). The positive impact of passively listening to uplifting music on positive emotion is also supported in the research (Campion & Levita, 2014; Sergeant & Mongrain, 2011). Campion and Levita (2014) saw gains in verbal fluency in participants who listened to uplifting music. The evidence suggests that listening to and practising music can support improvements in creativity.

Furthermore, listening to uplifting music (even for as little as a few minutes) reportedly decreased general physical symptoms of stress (Sergeant & Mongrain, 2011) and fatigue (Campion & Levita, 2014). The effect of music is so powerful that patients undergoing spinal surgery required less anaesthesia when listening to music (Koelsch et al., 2011). Thus, music offers an effective protection from pain. Furthermore, engaging in a music-listening intervention for 1 month resulted in a significant decrease in blood pressure, heart rate, respiratory rate, and depression (Chan et al., 2009). The physiological effect extends to brain functioning, meaning that music changes the function of the prefrontal cortex associated with decision-making, emotional regulation, and resilience (Arjmand et al., 2017). Therefore, a simple process of listening to music is associated with a range of positive outcomes.

Caveats

It is essential to match the activity with your personality style and activity type preference. For example, Sergeant and Mongrain's (2011) study showed no positive effects of listening to uplifting music for people who prefer having company to independent activities. So if you prefer to spend time with others, you may choose to select a different tool from this book to help you enhance your wellbeing. You might also bother your neighbours if the music is loud, which could ultimately impact your positive relationships.

References

Arjmand, H.-A., Hohagen, J., Paton, B., & Rickard, N. S. (2017). Emotional responses to music: Shifts in frontal brain asymmetry mark periods of musical change. *Frontiers in Psychology, 8*. https://doi-org.elib.tcd.ie/10.3389/fpsyg.2017.02044

Bernardi, L., Sleight, P., Bandinelli, G., Cencettin, S., Fattorini, L., Wdowczyc-Szulc, J., & Lagi, A. (2001). Effect of rosary prayer and yoga mantras on autonomic cardiovascular rhythms: Comparative study. *British Medical Journal, 323*, 22–29.

Campion, M., & Levita, L. (2014). Enhancing positive affect and divergent thinking abilities: Play some music and dance. *The Journal of Positive Psychology, 9*(2), 137–145. doi:10.1080/17439760.2013.848376

Chan, M. F., Chan, E. A., Mok, E., & Tse, F. Y. K. (2009). Effect of music on depression levels and physiological responses in community-based older adults. *International Journal of Mental Health Nursing, 18*(4), 285–294. https://doi-org.elib.tcd.ie/10.1111/j.1447-0349.2009.00614.x

Conner, T. S., DeYoung, C. G., & Silvia, P. J. (2018). Everyday creative activity as a path to flourishing. *The Journal of Positive Psychology, 13*(2), 181–189. doi:10.1080/17439760.2016.1257049

Croom, A. M. (2015). Music practice and participation for psychological wellbeing: A review of how music influences positive emotion, engagement, relationships, meaning, and accomplishment. *Musicae Scientiae, 19*(1), 44–64. https://doi.org/10.1177/1029864914561709

Koelsch, S., Fuermetz, J., Sack, U., Bauer, K., Hohenadel, M., Wiegel, M., Kaisers, U. X., & Heinke, W. (2011). Effects of music listening on cortisol levels and propofol consumption during spinal anesthesia. *Frontiers in Psychology, 2*. https://doi-org.elib.tcd.ie/10.3389/fpsyg.2011.00058

Ribeiro, F. S., Santos, F. H., Albuquerque, P. B., & Oliveira-Silva, P. (2019). Emotional induction through music: Measuring cardiac and electrodermal responses of emotional states and their persistence. *Frontiers in Psychology, 10*. https://doi-org.elib.tcd.ie/10.3389/fpsyg.2019.00451

Sergeant, S., & Mongrain, M. (2011). Are positive psychology exercises helpful for people with depressive personality styles? *The Journal of Positive Psychology, 6*(4), 260–272. doi:10.1080/17439760.2011.577089

Sharda, M., Tuerk, C., Chowdhury, R., Jamey, K., Foster, N., Custo-Blanch, M., Tan, M., Nadig, A., & Hyde, K. (2018). Music improves social communication and auditory-motor connectivity in children with autism. *Translational Psychiatry, 8*(1), 231. https://doi.org/10.1038/s41398-018-0287-3

Art viewing

Each year, as many as 10 million people visit the Louvre in Paris, France, to experience art. Leonardo da Vinci's *Salvador Mundi* sold for almost 500 million euros in 2017. So what is it about art that draws us to it? There are differences between experts and novices in how they experience art (Silvia, 2013). Experts tend to be less confused about the art they view and appreciate its aesthetics much more than novices. They also report experiencing different emotional reactions and are impacted by the new art differently. While novices are searching for paintings they recognise, for example, *Mona Lisa* in the Louvre (hence the queue to see it), experts become more interested in art when they find some novel art. Art viewing has long been perceived as a source of cognitive, emotional, and social satisfaction (Roberts et al., 2011). Although the preferences for art styles are different, some people prefer art galleries; others get a boost from viewing street art, such as graffiti (Mason et al., 2006). The beauty of art is that there is something in it for everyone. A recent scoping review of over 3,000 studies carried out by the World Health Organisation identified strong evidence for art viewing and art making being beneficial in preventing illness improving health and wellbeing (Fancourt & Finn, 2019). So why not give it a try?

Research-based tools

Tool 68: Lunchtime visit (Clow, 2006)

Pop into your local gallery for 30 minutes during your lunchtime. If you are like most of the participants in this study, your lunchtime visit may help you reduce your stress and enhance your wellbeing.

Tool 69: Digital art (adapted from Zubala et al., 2021)

You don't need to visit a gallery to benefit from art. Viewing art on your digital devices (e.g. laptop, tablet, phone) can effectively enhance your wellbeing. It also allows you to "visit" virtual galleries worldwide and enjoy a wide range of exhibitions.

Variation of practice

A visit to the art gallery can be used to increase empathy. Sherman and colleagues (2020) instructed visitors to take the perspective of the American Indian people depicted in the photographs. They found that taking the perspective of the other improved empathy levels. If you are into arts, you can extend your practice by reading about the paintings, organising physical or digital guides that will tell you the history behind each painting. You can pick and choose a variety of art types or architecture and observe their impact on you. Some may boost your positive emotions significantly; others might do it to a lesser extent. Until you try it, you will never know. Finally, some people enjoy art on their home and workplace walls. The pieces may be reproductions or just pretty paintings that bring joy into their lives.

Mental and physical health benefits

A recent review by Cotter and Pawelski (2022) described many benefits of visiting art galleries, including feeling restored, increased wellbeing, and feeling socially connected to others (when the visit was with other people). In addition, visiting art museums have been reported to increase positive emotion (Herron & Jamieson, 2020; Michalos & Kahlke, 2010; Thomson et al., 2018) and reduce anxiety, although the perceived anxiety levels differed (Binnie, 2010).

In terms of physiological health, Cotter and Pawelski's review (2022) describes research showing that visiting art museums reduces cortisol levels, suggesting a moderating effect on stress. Furthermore, there is evidence that it supports flourishing and health (Cotter & Pawelski, 2022). In one of the studies, office workers in London were asked to visit an art gallery for just 35 minutes on their lunch break (Clow & Fredhoi, 2006). The researchers tested the workers' cortisol levels before and after the gallery visit and saw a significant drop. They concluded that this brief visit amplified participants' recovery from the stress of their jobs.

Furthermore, researchers asked almost 400 people to wear electronic gloves as they visited a gallery (Tschacher et al., 2012). They measured participants' experience by gathering data about their heart rate and skin conductance response. They found that as they visited a gallery, each painting they looked at evoked different emotions and reactions in people, which in turn affected their cardiovascular health.

Visiting a gallery has also been used as part of the recovery process for people who experienced psychosis (Colbert et al., 2013). As part of their visit, they reflected on paintings and their meaning relative to their personal lives. It also showed a boost of wellbeing for patients with dementia and their carers (Johnson et al., 2017). Furthermore, in an experimental study conducted with patients with cancer who were recovering from major oncologic surgery, a visit to the hospital gallery had little effect on their pain threshold; however, it reduced their anxiety, and improved their hope and their overall mental wellbeing scores, all of which were helpful in their recovery (Lone et al., 2021). Thus, a simple activity of visiting a gallery is filled with a range of benefits.

Caveat

If you are not very familiar with visiting art museums, it may not reduce your anxiety to the same degree as for a regular visitor (Binnie, 2010). It's important to feel comfortable in the space, so maybe try a few times before you decide if it is for you or not.

References

Binnie, J. (2010). Does viewing art in the museum reduce anxiety and improve wellbeing? *Museums & Social Issues*, *5*(2), 191–201. https://doi.org/10.1179/msi.2010.5.2.191

Clow, A., & Fredhoi, C. (2006). Normalisation of salivary cortisol levels and self-report stress by a brief lunchtime visit to an art gallery by London City workers. *Journal of Holistic Healthcare*, *3*(2), 29–32.

Colbert, S., Cooke, A., Camic, P. M., & Springham, N. (2013). The art-gallery as a resource for recovery for people who have experienced psychosis. *The Arts in Psychotherapy*, *40*(2), 250–256. https://doi-org.elib.tcd.ie/10.1016/j.aip.2013.03.003

Cotter, Katherine N., & Pawelski, James O. (2022). Art museums as institutions for human flourishing. *The Journal of Positive Psychology*, *17*(2), 288–302, doi:10.1080/17439760.2021.2016911

Fancourt, D., & Finn, S. (2019). *What is the evidence on the role of the arts in improving health and wellbeing? A scoping review*. World Health Organization. Regional Office for Europe. https://apps.who.int/iris/handle/10665/329834. License: CC BY-NC-SA 3.0 IGO.

Herron, A., & Jamieson, A. (2020). Grandfathers at Melbourne Museum: Shining a spotlight on overlooked museum visitors. *Visitor Studies*, *23*(2), 101–119. https://doi.org/10.1080/10645578.2020.1772616

Johnson, J., Culverwell, A., Hulbert, S., Robertson, M., & Camic, P. M. (2017). Museum activities in dementia care: Using visual analog scales to measure subjective wellbeing. *Dementia* (14713012), *16*(5), 591–610. https://doi-org.elib.tcd.ie/10.1177/1471301215611763

Lone, Z., Hussein, A. A., Khan, H., Steele, M., Jing, Z., Attwood, K., Lin-Hill, J., Davidson, R., & Guru, K. A. (2021). Art heals: Randomized controlled study investigating the effect of a dedicated in-house art gallery on the recovery of patients after major oncologic surgery. *Annals of Surgery*, *274*(2), 264–270. https://doi-org.elib.tcd.ie/10.1097/SLA.0000000000004059

Mason, D. D. M., & McCarthy, C. (2006). 'The feeling of exclusion': Young peoples' perceptions of art galleries. *Museum Management & Curatorship*, *21*(1), 20–31. https://doi-org.elib.tcd.ie/10.1080/09647770600402101

Michalos, A. C., & Kahlke, P. M. (2010). Arts and perceived quality of life in British Colombia. *Social Indicators Research*, *96*(1), 1–39. https://doi.org/10.1007/s11205-009-9466-1

Roberts, S., Camic, P. M., & Springham, N. (2011). New roles for art galleries: Art-viewing as a community intervention for family carers of people with mental health problems. *Arts & Health: An International Journal of Research, Policy and Practice*, *3*(2), 146–159. https://doi-org.elib.tcd.ie/10.1080/17533015.2011.561360

Sherman, A., Cupo, L., Mithlo, N. M., & Eisenbarth, H. (2020). Perspective-taking increases emotionality and empathy but does not reduce harmful biases against American Indians: Converging evidence from the museum and lab. *Public Library of Science One*, *15*(2), e0228784. https://doi.org/10.1371/journal.pone.0228784

Silvia, P. J. (2013). Interested experts, confused novices: Art expertise and the knowledge emotions. *Empirical Studies of the Arts*, *31*(1), 107–115. https://doi.org/10.2190/EM.31.1.f

Thomson, L. J., Lockyer, B., Camic, P. M., & Chatterjee, H. J. (2018). Effects of a museum-based social prescription intervention on quantitative measures of psychological wellbeing in older adults. *Perspectives in Public Health*, *138*(1), 28–38. https://doi.org/10.1177/ 1757913917737563

Tschacher, W., Greenwood, S., Kirchberg, V., Wintzerith, S., van den Berg, K., & Tröndle, M. (2012). Physiological correlates of aesthetic perception of artworks in a museum. *Psychology of Aesthetics, Creativity, and the Arts*, *6*(1), 96–103. https://doi-org.elib.tcd.ie/10.1037/a0023845

Zubala, A., Kennell, N., & Hackett, S. (2021). Art therapy in the digital world: An integrative review of current practice and future directions. *Frontiers in Psychology*, *12*, 595536. https://doi-org.elib.tcd.ie/10.3389/fpsyg.2021.600070

Your reflection space

Which feeling-good tools would you like to try? Why?
Which activities did you find most useful? How did you tweak them?

6 Meaning-making tools

Life meaning is about helping us comprehend the world around us, consistency in understanding ourselves, and a clear life purpose (Steger et al., 2015). It is about understanding the world's complexities and how we fit into it. This comprehension results in higher life satisfaction and wellbeing. Thus, having life meaning provides a buffer against life stressors and a platform for thriving.

The research associated with life meaning takes three distinct routes (Steger, 2009):

1 Presence of meaning
2 Sources of meaning
3 Search for meaning

Research on meaning tries to identify who has life meaning and who doesn't. Furthermore, it explores the sources of life meaning and identifies what makes life more meaningful or what we draw from to make it more meaningful. Finally, research on the search for meaning tries to identify the process and outcomes of finding out what our life meaning is. Those who search for meaning feel that their lives are meaningless, which causes them further distress. In contrast, some make it their life mission to find meaning in life, and their search does not upset them to the same extent. Thus, people differ in how the search of meaning impacts them.

In this section, we will delve into tools that will help you find general life meaning and support you in discovering the meaning of suffering we experience in our lives.

The meaning-making tools include:

1 Exploring meaning
2 Positive identity
3 Benefit finding

DOI: 10.4324/9781003279594-8

4 Legacy
5 Photography

References

Steger, M., Fitch-Martin, A., Donnelly, J., & Rickard, K. (2015). Meaning in life and health: Proactive health orientation links meaning in life to health variables among American undergraduates. *Journal of Happiness Studies*, *16*, 583–597.

Steger, M. (2009). Meaning. In S. Lopez (Ed.), *Encyclopaedia of positive psychology* (pp. 605–609). Wiley Blackwell.

Exploring meaning

Victor Frankl (1997, 2000) was a psychiatrist who spent years during World War II as a prisoner of the Nazis in a concentration camp. During his ordeal, he observed many prisoners lose hope at the early stages of imprisonment, whereas others kept going, kept hoping, kept fighting against the oppressors. After the war, some people thrived, whereas others found it challenging to live everyday life. What was different between these two groups boiled down to one thing: having life meaning. Following his discovery, he created a new therapeutic approach called logotherapy. This therapy is unlike others in that it is not focused on enhancing wellbeing or reducing depression. Instead, it is focused on discovering life meaning. Frankl found that once former prisoners of war became aware of the meaning of their suffering, their lives were transformed. However, it took some of them years to figure it out, while others accomplished it in one therapeutic session. Based on the principles of logotherapy, Wong (2012) proposed the PURE model as an adaptation of logotherapy and a pathway to help people go through the process of discovering their life meaning.

Research-based tools

Tool 70: Logotherapy (adapted from Devoe, 2012)

According to Logotherapy, there are three ways in which meaning of life can be discovered:

1 Creative value – Try to reflect on what work or task you can create to add value with and how your experience allowed you to develop as a person and what you can give back to the society.
2 Experiential value – Consider what you have received that you value, are grateful for and appreciate in life.

3 Attitudinal value – Suffering in life is inevitable. Reflect on what attitude can help you embrace it.

Tool 71: PURE model (adapted from Wong, 2012)

You can follow the PURE principles on your own or do it with a therapist or a coach. PURE is an acronym for (1) purpose, (2) understanding, (3) responsibility, (4) enjoyment. You can either reflect on each part of the model or write down your responses.

> **Purpose** – what is your direction in life? What is your passion? What do you value most? Which parts of who you are do you accept? What helps you experience positive emotions? What have you done that helped you feel accomplished?
> **Understanding** – what narratives that you tell yourself about your life help or hinder you? What is your belief system? How do you describe yourself? How realistic is your positive thinking about life?
> **Responsibility** – what do you do that helps you live as a good person? When you did the right thing, what was it? In what way are you engaged in civic virtues? What do you do to fulfil your potential?
> **Enjoyment** – how do you feel about your life? Do you have higher levels of wellbeing? If not, what can you do to enhance your wellbeing? What aspects of your life are you satisfied with?

Tool 72: Life crafting (adapted from Schippers & Ziegler, 2019)

Reflect and make progress on the following:

1 Discover your values in life (what is important to you) and your passions (what keeps you interested).
2 Reflect on your competencies (what you can do well) and habits, both existing and aspirational
3 Reflect on your social life, both your current life and the life you desire to have.
4 Reflect on your desired and potential future career.
5 Sit down and, over the next 20 minutes, write down about your ideal future. Repeat this exercise daily or weekly if needed.
6 Write down your goal and plan for obstacles. When they happen, what will you do?
7 Tell your family and friends about the goals you've set up for yourself. This public commitment will provide you with more social support and help you become more motivated.

Variations of practice

Try to figure out what matters in life for you, and like a child, keep asking: why does it matter? Over and over again, until you get to the bottom of why the things you believe are essential to you are indeed vital.

Check out other tools in this book

Reminiscence tool is also a powerful medium for meaning making.

Mental and physical health benefits

Even though the main objective of logotherapy is to enhance life meaning, which is a deeper level of wellbeing (eudemonic), many studies showed that engaging in the logotherapy process boosts subjective and psychological wellbeing in adults and younger people (e.g. Faramarzi & Bavali, 2017; Liu et al., 2021), as well as reduces depression (e.g. Baumel Constantino, 2020; Kim & Choi, 2021). In addition to this, it effectively reduced demoralisation in women with gynaecological cancer (Fan-Ko et al., 2021). Also, the quality of life and the severity of symptoms of the irritable bowel syndrome declined following logotherapy sessions (Taghlidabad & Mashhadi, 2020). Furthermore, even though the therapy was not designed as an end-of-life practice, several studies showed that this meaning-making therapy was helpful for patients in palliative care (Breitbart et al., 2004).

The life crafting activity focuses on reflecting what is important to us, and a significant part of it delves into our meaning in the context of work. Following a lifelong longitudinal study that followed participants from 17 to 20 years old until they died, Vaillant (2002) observed that a career developed in midlife that will allow individuals to contribute to society is crucial to ensure positive ageing. When we skip our career development stage, we find it harder, later on, to engage in the generativity stage of our lives, which refers to leaving our mark on the younger generation, contributing to the society and the world we will be leaving behind when we die. We've had just one career, which was a job for life in the past. Nowadays, however, we have several careers throughout our lives, and since we live much longer than we used to, we often have a career past our retirement. Thus, it is never too late to learn and dream of what we want to do "when we grow up".

Caveats

Finding meaning in life is one of the most challenging endeavours you can take on. Beware that the search for meaning is associated with lower levels of wellbeing. Therefore, if you are in a situation in which you do not know your life meaning, the journey of discovery may be challenging. You may need help with this in the form of working with coaches or therapists. If your wellbeing is very low, this activity may not be suitable for you if you were to do it on your own.

References

Baumel, W. T., & Constantino, J. N. (2020). Implementing logotherapy in its second half-century: Incorporating existential considerations into personalized treatment of adolescent depression. *Journal of the American Academy of Child & Adolescent Psychiatry*, 59(9), 1012–1015. https://doi-org.elib.tcd.ie/10.1016/j.jaac.2020.06.006

Breitbart, W., Gibson, C., Poppito, S. R., & Berg, A. (2004). Psychotherapeutic interventions at the end of life: A focus on meaning and spirituality. *The Canadian Journal of Psychiatry/La Revue Canadienne de Psychiatrie*, 49(6).

Devoe, D. (2012). Viktor Frankl's logotherapy: The search for purpose and meaning. *Inquiries Journal*, 4(07).

Fan-Ko Sun, Chao-Ming Hung, YuChun Yao, Chi-Feng Fu, Pei-Jung Tsai, & Chun-Ying Chiang. (2021). The effects of logotherapy on distress, depression, and demoralization in breast cancer and gynecological cancer patients: A preliminary study. *Cancer Nursing*, 44(1), 53–61. https://doi-org.elib.tcd.ie/10.1097/NCC.0000000000000740

Faramarzi, S., & Bavali, F. (2017). The effectiveness of group logotherapy to improve psychological wellbeing of mothers with intellectually disabled children. *International Journal of Developmental Disabilities*, 63(1), 45–51. https://doi-org.elib.tcd.ie/10.1080/20473869.2016.1144298

Frankl, V. (2000). *Man's search for ultimate meaning*. MJF Books.

Frankl, V. E. (1997). *Man's search for ultimate meaning*. Insight Books/Plenum Press.

Kim, C., & Choi, H. (2021). The efficacy of group logotherapy on community-dwelling older adults with depressive symptoms: A mixed methods study. *Perspectives in Psychiatric Care*, 57(2), 920–928. https://doi-org.elib.tcd.ie/10.1111/ppc.12635

Liu, C., McCabe, M., Dawson, A., Cyrzon, C., Shankar, S., Gerges, N., Kellett-Renzella, S., Chye, Y., & Cornish, K. (2021). Identifying predictors of university students' wellbeing during the COVID-19 pandemic-A data-driven approach. *International Journal of Environmental Research and Public Health*, 18(13). https://doi-org.elib.tcd.ie/10.3390/ijerph18136730

Schippers, M. C., & Ziegler, N. (2019). Life crafting as a way to find purpose and meaning in life. *Frontiers in Psychology*, 10, 2778. https://doi.org/10.3389/fpsyg.2019.02778

Taghlidabad, B. G., & Mashhadi, R. T. (2020). The effects of group logotherapy on the severity of irritable bowel syndrome and the quality of life of the affected patients. *Journal of Practice in Clinical Psychology*, 8(1), 39–46.

Vaillant, G. E. (2002). *Aging well: surprising guideposts to a happier life from the landmark study of adult development*. Little Brown.

Wong, P. (2012). From logotherapy to meaning-centred counselling and therapy. In Paul T. P. Wong (Ed.), *The human quest for meaning: Theories, research, and applications* (2nd ed., pp. 619–647). Routledge/Taylor & Francis Group.

Positive identity

How you view yourself will impact your outcomes, as it becomes a self-fulfilling prophecy guiding your life choices. Your identity refers to unique attributes from others, such as your traits, strengths, and aspects of your physical self. These attributes may be either negative or positive. Similarly, your social identity refers to your attributes related to your social group membership. Belonging to a group helps individuals maintain or enhance aspects of their identity. Belonging to a group is particularly important for individuals who feel stigmatised, e.g. performing specific jobs that can either improve your self-image or make you feel worse about yourself; weight – seeing yourself as too thin or too big; appearance; being a cancer or heart attack survivor; belonging to an ethnic, disability, or sexual minority. Group belonging can help us overcome the negative view of self and embrace what is unique about us more positively.

Given that the negative is much stronger than the positive (Baumeister et al., 2001), our negatives are much more accessible than the positives. Importantly, when we suffer from a chronic illness, it can become part of our identity for better or worse. Van Bulck et al. (2018) explain that our identity about a chronic illness can move between feeling engulfed and wanting to reject the illness identity and, on the positive side, to acceptance and even feeling enriched by the experience of the illness. Therefore, activities associated with positive identity help us draw a more balanced perspective on who we are and notice both positives and negatives about ourselves.

This section will delve into self-identity and social identity as tools for making meaning of who we are.

Research-based tools

Tool 73: Social identity–based self-affirmation (adapted from Ball & Nario-Redmond, 2014)

- Join a group that reaffirms your identity, e.g. if you are vegan, join a vegan group; if you love knitting, join a knitting group.
- Identify the positive characteristics of a group to which you feel you belong and identify which characteristics are associated with you,

e.g. cancer survivors are courageous, strong, empowered, and fighters; runners preparing for a marathon are persistent, hardworking, eat healthy.
- Redefining personal identity based on the social identity, e.g. I hike regularly, I'm a hiker, meaning I love being in nature; I like dancing, I'm a dancer, meaning I'm into rhythm and soul.
- Practicing self-affirmation is whereby you begin to describe yourself and self-stereotype positively based on your group belonging, e.g. I'm a smart geek that loves reading and doesn't care about being called boring; I'm a night-clubber; I love dressing up and having fun.

Tool 74: Positive introduction (adapted from Rashid & Seligman, 2019)

Write down a page about a time when you have managed a tricky situation very well. It doesn't need to be a life-changing event. Instead, write a story of how this event got the best out of you. What personal (e.g. optimism, faith) or environmental (e.g. support from friends, organisations) attributes helped you handle this situation so well? How has this story become part of who you are, or how can it become your new self-concept in the future?

Please note that this tool has been assessed as part of Positive Psychotherapy (Rashid, 2015), not a stand-alone intervention.

Tool 75: Best possible self in the present (adapted from Carrillo et al., 2021)

Sit down and visualise your best possible self as you are today. Consider your abilities (what you do well), your assets (qualities of your character, strengths) that you perceive as most relevant in the context of the best version of yourself.

Variations of practice

You can re-define and self-affirm positive social identities through group discussions with people belonging to that group and others who perceive it positively. To add to the positive introduction, you can write an introduction using your character strengths. One of our clients has taken this idea further and re-wrote his CV (without sending it to anyone). Instead of accomplishments associated with job progress, he mentioned his personal accomplishments, how he had overcome adversity and used and developed his strengths in all his jobs. Taking his lead on it, you can do the same about any aspect of your life. Suppose you are trying to figure out your identity relating to dating. In that case, you may go through reviewing all your relationships and identifying what you have learnt from them, what strengths you have used, and what methods helped you overcome challenges. Whilst these activities have not yet been tested empirically, if they feel suitable for you, why not give them a try?

Mental and physical health benefits

Social identity interventions have a moderate to substantial impact on health (Steffens et al., 2021). Identification with a group, in other words, "owning" your identity and your uniqueness and going as far as self-stereotyping, e.g. I'm gay; therefore I do x; I'm African American; consequently, I do y, is associated with higher levels of wellbeing and life satisfaction (Latrofoa et al., 2009; Sani et al., 2010). It is also associated with improved physical health and better immune system functioning (Ysseldyk et al., 2018). In transgender men and women, carrying out positive identity interventions is associated with higher levels of resilience (Amodeo et al., 2018) and wellbeing (Clements et al., 2021). In individuals with acquired brain injury, their quality of life improved when they re-defined who they were now as people (Wood, 2008).

Caveats

Affirming one's new identity, even if it is a positive identity, is also associated with losing the previous identity, which may cause mixed emotions. It is important to find social support before major identity changes occur. Also, seek out help from coaches and therapists when this process is becoming too challenging for you.

References

Amodeo, A. L., Picariello, S., Valerio, P., & Scandurra, C. (2018). Empowering transgender youths: Promoting resilience through a group training program. *Journal of Gay & Lesbian Mental Health*, 22(1), 3–19. https://doi.org/10.1080/19359705.2017.1361880

Ball, T. C., & Nario-Redmond, M. R. (2014). Positive social identity interventions: Finding a conduit for well-being in members of stigmatized groups. In A. C. Parks & S. M. Schueller (Eds.), *The Wiley-Blackwell handbook of positive psychological interventions* (pp. 327–343). Wiley-Blackwell.

Baumeister, R. F., Bratslavsky, E., Finkenauer, C., & Vohs, K. D. (2001). Bad is stronger than good. *Review of General Psychology*, 5(4), 323–370. https://doi.org/10.1037/1089-2680.5.4.323

Carrillo, A., Etchemendy, E., & Baños, R. M. (2021). My best self in the past, present or future: Results of two randomized controlled trials. *Journal of Happiness Studies*, *22*(2), 955–980. https://doi-org.elib.tcd.ie/10.1007/s10902-020-00259-z

Clements, Z. A., Rostosky, S. S., McCurry, S., & Riggle, E. D. B. (2021). Piloting a brief intervention to increase positive identity and wellbeing in transgender and nonbinary individuals. *Journal of Comparative Psychology*, *135*(2), 1. https://doi-org.elib.tcd.ie/10.1037/pro0000390

Latrofoa, M., Vaes, J., Pastore, M., & Cadinu, M. (2009). "United we stand, divided we fall"! The protective function of self-stereotyping for stigmatised members' psychological wellbeing. *Applied Psychology: An International Review*, *58*, 84–104.

Rashid, T. (2015). Positive psychotherapy: A strength-based approach. *The Journal of Positive Psychology*, *10*(1), 25–40. https://doi-org.elib.tcd.ie/10.1080/17439760.2014.920411

Rashid, T., & Seligman, M. E. P. (2019). *Positive psychotherapy: Workbook*. Oxford University Press.

Sani, F., Magrin, M. E., Scrignaro, M., & McCollum, R. (2010). Ingroup identification mediates the effects of subjective ingroup status on mental health. *British Journal of Social Psychology*, *49*, 8830983.

Steffens, N. K., LaRue, C. J., Haslam, C., Walter, Z. C., Cruwys, T., Munt, K. A., Haslam, S. A., Jetten, J., & Tarrant, M. (2021). Social identification-building interventions to improve health: A systematic review and meta-analysis. *Health Psychology Review*, *15*(1), 85–112. https://doi-org.elib.tcd.ie/10.1080/17437199.2019.1669481

Van Bulck, L., Goossens, E., Luyckx, K., Oris, L., Apers, S., & Moons, P. (2018). Illness identity: A novel predictor for healthcare use in adults with congenital heart disease. *Journal of the American Heart Association*, *7*(11), e008723. https://doi.org/10.1161/JAHA.118.008723

Wood, R. L. (2008). Long-term outcome of serious traumatic brain injury. *European Journal of Anaesthesiology*, *42*(Supplement), 115–122. https://doi.org/10.1017/S0265021507003432

Ysseldyk, R., McQuaid, R. J., McInnis, O. A., Anisman, H., & Matheson, K. (2018). The ties that bind: Ingroup ties are linked with diminished inflammatory immune responses and fewer mental health symptoms through less rumination. *PloS One*, *13*(4), e0195237. https://doi-org.elib.tcd.ie/10.1371/journal.pone.0195237

Benefit finding

Benefit finding is the ability to see the silver lining in the darkest clouds. Most people automatically search for benefits after stressful or traumatic events in their lives (Tennen & Affleck, 2005) or aim to see what could be even worse about their situation (Teigen & Jensen, 2011). Perceiving a benefit of a bad situation gives their suffering meaning. This is why it is often seen as one of the routes towards experiencing post-traumatic growth (PTG), which is a realisation that traumatic events resulted in one of the five positive outcomes:

1 Becoming closer to some people
2 Feeling you are stronger than you thought you were
3 Seeing new possibilities in life
4 Becoming more spiritual
5 Appreciating life more

In addition to these psychological symptoms of growth, some people experience corporeal post-traumatic growth (Hefferon, 2012), indicating the embodied growth after undergoing physical health issues, such as cancer, long COVID-19, heart attack, or stroke. Their growth is therefore associated with:

1 Having a new relationship with their body, being kinder to the body (e.g. not pushing yourself too hard when exercising) has gone through so much ordeal.
2 Increasing awareness of health and conscious health behaviour changes, which may result in improved nutrition or smoking cessation.
3 Building psychological resilience by making changes to your body using tools such as benefit finding can aid in accomplishing this.

Research-based tools

Tool 76: Benefit finding (adapted from King & Miner, 2000)

This tool may be helpful to anyone experiencing a traumatic or adverse event. Think back to an adverse or traumatic life event you've experienced, perhaps a loss of some sort that felt devastating to you. Consider the circumstances associated with this event. Now, refocus your attention on the positive aspects of this experience. Take a piece of paper, and for the next 20 minutes, write down the following:

- How has this experience benefitted you as a person?
- How has this event made you better equipped to cope with challenges in the future?

Don't worry about your spelling or grammar. Nobody is going to read this apart from you. So just let go, and go deep as you write about the benefits of the bad experience.

Tool 77: Benefit reminding (adapted from Tennen & Affleck, 2005)

This tool is useful for anyone going through chronic illness, like alcoholism, or experiencing ongoing pain. It encourages you to take time and remind yourself daily about the benefits of your chronic illness.

Tool 78: What might have been . . . (adapted from Kennedy et al., 2021)

This tool relates to imagining a negative situation in the context of how it might have been worse, in other words, what is the worst thing that could happen.

Tool 79: One door closes, another door opens (adapted from Gander et al., 2013)

Every day for the next week, reflect on the time when one door closed in your life (a negative event occurred), and soon after, another door opened (something positive happened to you as a result of the negative event).

This activity has been initially assessed as part of the positive psychotherapy programme (Rashid & Anjum, 2008).

Variations of practice

While most research focused on coping with bad news, one study identified the effect of the benefit-finding tool before receiving terrible news (Rankin & Sweeny, 2021). When people wait for critical news, e.g. exam or biopsy results, they may worry – so identifying a potential silver lining before the bad news helps you cope with the news and does not backfire when you receive positive news. Also, "reminding" yourself about the negative situation that occurred in the past and considering how it resulted in benefits can be just as beneficial as "finding" the benefits in a novel situation (Tennen & Affleck, 2005).

Mental and physical health benefits

A meta-analysis of benefit-finding activities showed that searching for benefits resulted in higher levels of wellbeing, quality of life, improved physical health, and a reduction in depression and anxiety (Helgeson et al., 2006). Activities such as benefit finding help with psychological adjustment, which is why they are instrumental when coping with challenges (Tennen & Affleck, 2005). Downward counterfactual thinking, which relates to the "It could have been worse" tool, is associated with higher levels of post-traumatic growth (Kennedy et al., 2021) and a more grateful disposition (Walsh & Egan, 2018).

Even though many therapists feel uncomfortable recommending this activity to their patients, benefit finding is a natural process for most of us when facing trauma. For example, in a study with people whose partners, children, or other family members were in hospice care, the researchers found that 6 months following the loss of their loved one, more than 70% of participants reported something positive, a benefit of their experience (Davis et al., 1998). Furthermore, those who could name a positive outcome of their horrendous situation were less distressed 7 months later. Therefore, the process of reflecting on the benefits of traumatic events helps us come to terms with our loss.

Benefit finding is a valuable tool helping patients make sense of their chronic illness (Pakenham, 2011). This also includes patients experiencing chronic mental health issues, whereby their ability to reflect on the benefits predicted the speed of their recovery (Chiba et al., 2011). It may be because chronic illness, unlike short-term illness, requires adjusting to the new way of life. Therefore, reflecting on the benefits of the situation helps us make the best out of a challenging situation. At the same time, according to a study with almost 7,000 cancer patients, the majority of them were able to find benefits in their situation (Liu et al., 2021).

Caveats

When considering "what might have been", it is essential to focus on the factors within your control. Otherwise, this tool may not be as effective. Also, beware of using this activity by considering the positive scenarios, i.e. all the good things you have missed out on, as they may result in you experiencing regret. Finally, beware of timing regarding the silver lining or benefit-finding activity. Whilst it is helpful to many people immediately after an adverse event, some may find it too upsetting to engage with. The "tyranny of positive thinking" should be avoided here, so please do not engage with this tool if it does not sit right with you at this moment in time. Finally, research with cancer patients is inconsistent about the benefits of this tool, as one study showed that it predicted patients to experience more negative emotions (Tomich & Helgeson, 2004); therefore, please use this activity with caution. If you are not ready for it, please leave it.

References

Chiba, R., Kawakami, N., & Miyamoto, Y. (2011). Quantitative relationship between recovery and benefit-finding among persons with chronic mental illness in Japan. *Nursing & Health Sciences*, *13*(2), 126–132. https://doi-org.elib.tcd.ie/10.1111/j.1442-2018.2011.00589.x

Davis, C. G., Nolen-Hoeksema, S., & Larson, J. (1998). Making sense of loss and benefiting from the experience: Two construals of meaning. *Journal of Personality and Social Psychology, 75*(2), 561–574. https://doi-org.elib.tcd.ie/10.1037/0022-3514.75.2.561

Gander, F., Proyer, R., Ruch, W., & Wyss, T. (2013). Strength-based positive interventions: Further evidence for their potential in enhancing well-being and alleviating depression. *Journal of Happiness Studies, 14*(4), 1241–1259.

Hefferon, K. (2012). Bring back the body into positive psychology: The theory of corporeal posttraumatic growth. *Psychology, 3*(12) 1238–1242.

Helgeson, V. S., Reynolds, K. A., & Tomich, P. L. (2006). A meta-analytic review of benefit finding and growth. *Journal of Consulting & Clinical Psychology, 74*(5), 797–816. https://doi-org.elib.tcd.ie/10.1037/0022-006X.74.5.797

Kennedy, C., Deane, F. P., & Chan, A. Y. C. (2021). "What might have been . . .": Counterfactual thinking, psychological symptoms and posttraumatic growth when a loved one is missing. *Cognitive Therapy & Research, 45*(2), 322–332. https://doi-org.elib.tcd.ie/10.1007/s10608-020-10156-7

King, L. A., & Miner, K. N. (2000). Writing about the perceived benefits of traumatic events: Implications for physical health. *Personality and Social Psychology Bulletin, 26*(2), 220–230. https://doi.org/10.1177/0146167200264008

Liu, Z., Thong, M. S. Y., Doege, D., Koch-Gallenkamp, L., Bertram, H., Eberle, A., Holleczek, B., Waldmann, A., Zeissig, S. R., Pritzkuleit, R., Brenner, H., & Arndt, V. (2021). Prevalence of benefit finding and posttraumatic growth in long-term cancer survivors: Results from a multi-regional population-based survey in Germany. *British Journal of Cancer, 125*(6), 877–883. https://doi-org.elib.tcd.ie/10.1038/s41416-021-01473-z

Pakenham, K. I. (2011). Benefit-finding and sense-making in chronic illness. In S. Folkman (Ed.), *The Oxford handbook of stress, health, and coping* (pp. 242–268). Oxford University Press.

Rankin, K., & Sweeny, K. (2021). Preparing silver linings for a cloudy day: The consequences of preemptive benefit finding. *Personality & Social Psychology Bulletin*, 1461672211037863. https://doi-org.elib.tcd.ie/10.1177/01461672211037863

Rashid, T., & Anjum, A. (2008). Positive psychotherapy for young adults and children. In J. R. Z. Abela & B. L. Hankin (Eds.), *Handbook of depression in children and adolescents* (pp. 250–287). The Guilford Press.

Teigen, K. H., & Jensen, T. K. (2011). Unlucky victims or lucky survivors? Spontaneous counterfactual thinking by families exposed to the tsunami disaster. *European Psychologist, 16*(1), 48–57. https://doi-org.elib.tcd.ie/10.1027/1016-9040/a000033

Tennen, H., & Affleck, G. (2005). Benefit-finding and benefit reminding. In C. R. Snyder & S. J. Lopez (Eds.), *Handbook of positive psychology* (pp. 584–597). Oxford University Press.

Tomich, P. L., & Helgeson, V. S. (2004). Is finding something good in the bad always good? Benefit finding among women with breast cancer. *Health Psychology, 23*(1), 16–23.

Walsh, N., & Egan, S. (2018). *Things could have been worse: The counterfactual nature of gratitude* (pp. 339–349). AICS.

Legacy (scarcity)

The wisdom of hindsight is something you may have already experienced, thus appreciating its value. This activity helps you reflect on it further and gain all the benefits of it ahead of time. It allows you to project yourself into the future (good or bad) and, from this perspective, choose to make decisions in the present about the changes you need to make to either avoid what you do not want to happen or find a pathway to achieve what you desire. It is a wake-up call for some and a motivator to embrace change without delay. It can potentially transform your life by delving deeper into what matters to you. The effect of these activities relates to the concept of scarcity.

Research-based tools

Tool 80: Most feared obituary (adapted from Frisch, 2006)

Imagine that you didn't manage to change all your unhealthy and unhappy behaviour patterns before your death. Review all your current habits and routines that make your life unhealthy and unhappy, and imagine what would happen if these problems got a worse year on year until you die. Imagine a long life and that you do not make any positive changes to the way you live it. Your standards, priorities and goals remain the same, and as you let yourself go, your happiness and health continue to deteriorate. Now, write your obituary. Make it very personal and detailed. Imagine your family, friends, and strangers will read it in the newspaper and online. Write about your life as it would be if you didn't change the unhealthy and unhappy ways you live.

Tool 81: Positive legacy (Rashid & Seligman, 2019)

Consider what you would like your life to be in the future and how you would like to be remembered by your family, friends, colleagues, and everyone else close to you. What would you like your legacy to be? What would you like them to say about you. Take 15 to 20 minutes to write it all down as you would like it to be.

Once you're finished, read it all back and make a plan for creating the legacy you've imagined. What changes do you need to make to your life today to make it happen? Set up goals to help you achieve those things and read it back regularly in the future.

Tool 82: Life summary review (adapted from Schueller, 2010)

Imagine you are a grandparent. Now, describe in detail how you would like your grandchildren to talk about you and your life. Write it down, and a few days later, review what you have written and list what changes you need to make in your life today to make it happen.

Tool 83: Temporal scarcity (adapted from Kurtz, 2008)

Imagine that you are moving away in 4 weeks. You are changing your neighbourhood, your city, or your country; you are leaving your home, and as such, you are leaving everyone and everything behind. What changes would you make in your life today, given that soon you will not be here anymore? What really matters to you?

Variations of practice

All these activities use the influence of scarcity to motivate us to reflect on what is essential in our lives, and as such, you can practice scarcity in all aspects of your life to get to the bottom of what matters. For example, when you find it difficult to motivate yourself to complete an educational programme, reflect on how little time you have left to graduate. Similarly, when you give a notice of termination at work, consider how little time you have left until you leave. What will you be missing out on when you leave?

Mental and physical health benefits

The Positive Legacy activity is part of a positive psychotherapy programme, whereas the Most Feared Obituary is part of the quality-of-life therapy. Both therapies provide evidence of effectiveness in enhancing health and wellbeing, reducing ill-being helping people experiencing chronic illness live a better life.

Positive psychotherapy was initially developed to help people with depression (Seligman et al., 2006) and has since been replicated in several randomised controlled trials, showing a significant decline in depression (e.g. Lü et al., 2013; Schueller & Parks, 2012). It has also been used effectively as part of a smoking cessation programme (Kahler et al., 2014) ad as a quality-of-life therapy for people with schizophrenia (Meyer et al., 2012), psychosis (Riches et al., 2016), and brain injury rehabilitation (Bertisch et al., 2014). Concerning physical health, it was helpful for people with diabetes (Celano, 2013) and cardiovascular disease (DuBois et al., 2012; Huffman et al., 2011). In the non-clinical population, several studies reported an increase in subjective and psychological wellbeing (Bolier et al., 2013).

Quality-of-life (QOL) therapy effectively reduces symptoms of depression (Grant et al., 1995) and increases positive emotions in patients with implantable cardioverter defibrillators (Carroll et al., 2020). It was reported useful for people waiting for liver transplants and as a quality-of-life (QoL) coaching (Frisch, 2013). Whilst the programme is extensive and the tool presented earlier is just one of many tools associated with it, many people find it useful.

Caveats

This tool is not appropriate for some people. We have heard clients say that it sends chills down their spine. Yet others found it exceptionally useful. Therefore, ensure you feel comfortable with it before you engage. Also, please note that "positive legacy" and "most feared obituary" come from well-researched therapies; however, they were tested only as part of the therapeutic approach, not on their own.

References

Bertisch, H., Rath, J., Long, C., Ashman, T., & Rashid, T. (2014). Positive psychology in rehabilitation medicine: A brief report. *NeuroRehabilitation*, *34*, 573–585.

Bolier, L., Haverman, M., Westerhof, G. J., Riper, H., Smit, F., & Bohlmeijer, E. (2013). Positive psychology interventions: A meta-analysis of randomized controlled studies. *BMC Public Health*, *13*, 119.10.1186/1471-2458-13-119

Carroll, A. J., Christon, L. M., Rodrigue, J. R., Fava, J. L., Frisch, M. B., & Serber, E. R. (2020). Implementation, feasibility, and acceptability of quality of life therapy to improve positive emotions among patients with implantable cardioverter defibrillators. *Journal of Behavioral Medicine*, *43*(6), 968–978. https://doi-org.elib.tcd.ie/10.1007/s10865-020-00153-2

Celano, C. M., Beale, E. E., Moore, S. V., Wexler, D. J., & Huffman, J. C. (2013). Positive psychological characteristics in diabetes: A review. *Current Diabetes Reports*, *13*, 917–929. doi:10.1007/s11892-013-0430-8

DuBois, C. M., Beach, S. R., Kashdan, T. B., Nyer, M. B., Park, E. R., Celano, C. M., & Huffman, J. C. (2012). Positive psychological attributes and cardiac outcomes: Associations, mechanisms, and interventions. *Psychosomatics: Journal of Consultation and Liaison Psychiatry*, *53*, 303–318.10.1016/j.psym.2012.04.004

Frisch, M. B. (2006). *Quality of life therapy: Applying a life satisfaction approach to positive psychology and cognitive therapy.* John Wiley & Sons Ltd.

Frisch, M. B. (2013). Evidence-based well-being/positive psychology assessment and intervention with quality of life therapy and coaching and the quality of life inventory (QOLI). *Social Indicators Research*, *114*(2), 193–227.

Grant, G. M., Salcedo, V., Hynan, L. S., Frisch, M. B., & Puster, K. (1995). Effectiveness of quality of life therapy for depression. *Psychological Reports*, *76*(3 Pt 2), 1203–1208. https://doi-org.elib.tcd.ie/10.2466/pr0.1995.76.3c.1203

Huffman, J. C., Mastromauro, C. A., Boehm, J. K., Seabrook, R., Fricchione, G. L., Denninger, J. W., & Lyubomirsky, S. (2011). Development of a positive psychology intervention for patients with acute cardiovascular disease. *Heart International*, *6*(2), e14. https://doi.org/10.4081/hi.2011.e14

Kahler, C. W., Spillane, N. S., Day, A., Clerkin, E., Parks, A., Leventhal, A. M., & Brown, R. A. (2014). Positive psychotherapy for smoking cessation: Treatment development, feasibility, and preliminary results. *The Journal of Positive Psychology*, *9*, 19–29. doi:10.1080/17439760.2013.826716

Kurtz, J. L. (2008). Looking to the future to appreciate the present: The benefits of perceived temporal scarcity. *Psychological Science* (0956–7976), *19*(12), 1238–1241. https://doi-org.elib.tcd.ie/10.1111/j.1467-9280.2008.02231.x

Lü, W., Wang, Z., & Liu, Y. (2013). A pilot study on changes of cardiac vagal tone in individuals with low trait positive affect: The effect of positive psychotherapy. *International Journal of Psychophysiology*, *88*(2), 213–217. https://doi-org.elib.tcd.ie/10.1016/j.ijpsycho.2013.04.012

Meyer, P. S., Johnson, D. P., Parks, A., Iwanski, C., & Penn, D. L. (2012). Positive living: A pilot study of group positive psychotherapy for people with schizophrenia. *The Journal of Positive Psychology*, *7*, 239–248. doi:10.1080/17439760.2012.677467

Rashid, T., & Seligman, M. E. P. (2019). *Positive psychotherapy: Workbook*. Oxford University Press.

Riches, S., Schrank, B., Rashid, T., & Slade, M. (2016). WELLFOCUS PPT: Modifying positive psychotherapy for psychosis. *Psychotherapy*, *53*(1), 68–77. https://doi-org.elib.tcd.ie/10.1037/pst0000013

Schueller, S. M. (2010). Preferences for positive psychology exercises. *The Journal of Positive Psychology*, *5*(3), 192–203. https://doi.org/10.1080/17439761003790948

Schueller, S. M., & Parks, A. C. (2012). Disseminating self-help: Positive psychology exercises in an online trial. *Journal of Medical Internet Research*, *14*(3), 8–18. https://doi-org.elib.tcd.ie/10.2196/jmir.1850

Seligman, M. E. P., Rashid, T., & Parks, A. C. (2006). Positive psychotherapy. *The American Psychologist*, *61*(8), 774–788. https://doi-org.elib.tcd.ie/10.1037/0003-066X.61.8.774

Photography

An adage tells us that a picture is worth a thousand words. It has a unique ability to reflect our thoughts and feelings in a single image. Some of the most famous photographs in history not only captured moments in time, but they have also communicated to the world a deep meaning of these moments. That meaning stayed with us, not necessarily the picture's composition. For example, the iconic photograph of a soldier embracing and kissing a dental nurse in Times Square taken in 1945 by Alfred Eisenstaedt became a symbol of the joyous end of the atrocities of the war and the common folk's lives returning to normal. Another photograph, a picture of then Fidel Castro's associate, Che Guevara, taken by Alberto Corda, became the symbol of freedom or aggression, depending on our

Meaning-making tools 147

viewpoint. Today, we still see graffiti of Che worldwide, and some people wear T-shirts bearing his image. As controversial as his character is, the meaning we derive from the picture goes deeper than his face. After all, an image is not just an image; it is a symbol, which is sometimes worth a thousand words. This is why the researchers have used photographs to help us understand our life meaning, which this tool is all about.

Research-based tools

Tool 84: Through the windows of the soul (adapted from Steger et al., 2014)

Take a camera or have your smartphone camera ready, and for the next week, take 9 to 12 photographs of what gives your life meaning. Then, a week later, reflect on each photograph taken and write down what it represents and why you believe it makes your life meaningful.

Tool 85: Meaningful moments (adapted from Van Zyl et al., 2019)

Take a photograph a day and share it, unfiltered, on social media, such as Instagram. Describe briefly to your followers what makes each photograph meaningful for you.

Tool 86: Picture this! (adapted from McKee et al., 2019)

Over the next 21 days, catch yourself during the moments when you experience positive emotions. Using your smartphone, take a picture of each moment. Every evening, review all the pictures of the positive moments you have taken. Then, once a week, share the pictures and discuss them in person with your family and friends.

Variations of practice

Whilst the Steger et al. (2014) experiment used a maximum of 12 photographs, you can vary the number of photographs you take and describe. Also, instead of searching for a photo that depicts your life meaning, you may choose to spend a few hours reviewing your past photographs and selecting the meaningful moments from them. In addition to Instagram, you may use a different social media platform or share your photos in a closed group via WhatsApp, ChatWe, or something similar. Finally, given that the social impact is so significant, feel free to discuss some of the pictures with your friends and family for a potentially more powerful effect, ideally face to face over a cup of tea or your favourite beverage.

Mental and physical health benefits

In the first photo-ethnography research, the tool significantly improved participants' meaning in life and life satisfaction and boosted their experiences of positive emotions (Steger et al., 2014). In a similar study that involved sharing the photographs via Instagram, participants' life satisfaction has improved along with their presence of meaning (Van Zyl et al., 2019). The Picture This! research reported not only improvements of daily experiences of positive emotions, but having a day filled with joyous moments predicted enhanced levels of wellbeing the next day (McKee et al., 2019). Furthermore, participants in both the experimental and control groups experienced improved overall self-reported health. Therefore, doing something for their wellbeing, regardless of how small, may have had this effect on them. Finally, the impact of photography on the clinical population varies (Buchan, 2020). Some participants reported a significant improvement in functioning, while it was ineffective for others. However, this activity was also influential in making sense and finding meaning in their illness.

Caveats

Keep in mind why you are doing this activity. You are not trying to take perfect photographs; you are not doing it for other people; instead, you are doing it to help you clarify your life meaning. This is why you mustn't put any additional pressure on yourself by raising your expectations about the quality of your pictures. Please note that this tool is not beneficial for everyone.

References

Buchan, C. A. (2020). Therapeutic benefits and limitations of participatory photography for adults with mental health problems: A systematic search and literature review. *Journal of Psychiatric & Mental Health Nursing* (John Wiley & Sons, Inc.), 27(5), 657–668. https://doi-org.elib.tcd.ie/10.1111/jpm.12606

McKee, L. G., Algoe, S. B., Faro, A. L., O'Leary, J. L., & O'Neal, C. W. (2019). Picture this! Bringing joy into focus and developing healthy habits of mind: Rationale, design, and implementation of a randomized control trial for young adults. *Contemporary Clinical Trials Communications*, 15, 100391. https://doi-org.elib.tcd.ie/10.1016/j.conctc.2019.100391

Steger, M. F., Shim, Y., Barenz, J., & Shin, J. Y. (2014). Through the windows of the soul: A pilot study using photography to enhance meaning in life. *Journal of Contextual Behavioral Science*, *3*(1), 27–30. https://doiorg.elib.tcd.ie/10.1016/j.jcbs.2013.11.002

Van Zyl, L. E., Hulshof, I., & Dickens, L. R. (2019). #NoFilter: An online photographic meaningful-moments intervention. In L. E. Van Zyl & S. Rothmann Sr. (Eds.), *Evidence-based positive psychological interventions in multi-cultural contexts* (pp. 57–82). Springer Nature Switzerland AG. https://doi-org.elib.tcd.ie/10.1007/978-3-030-20311-5_3

Your reflection space

Which meaning-making tools would you like to try? Why?
Which activities did you find most useful? How did you tweak them?

7 Relationship tools

Suppose someone asked us which group of interventions makes the most significant difference to our wellbeing; we would easily say it is relationships. Positive relationships are one component of wellbeing included in all the flourishing/wellbeing models (Burke, 2021). Some researchers disagree about including positive emotions; others do not consider accomplishment important. But one thing they all include is relationships. Positive relationships relate to the support we give and receive from others and how we nurture that in our lives. One of the co-founders of positive psychology famously said "people matter", as he considered the people in our lives quintessential to life worthwhile living.

In their latest book, Prilleltensky and Prilleltensky (2021) describe the need we all have to matter. The authors argue that all the bad things that happen in our lives and society derive from this simple yet profound need to matter. For example, when the relationship with our loved ones goes off track, we act out because we want to matter. Likewise, when political movements with radical ideas take over, the minority of people want to feel like they matter. Therefore, according to the authors, in our relationships with others, we need to feel valued and feel like we add value regardless of how distant they are. Until this happens, we will struggle and act out to ensure we are listened to and feel we matter. This chapter will review tools that will help you nurture relationships with others in which you both feel you matter.

The relationship tools include:

1   Capitalisation
2   Forgiveness
3   Kindness
4   Savouring relationships

References

Burke, J. (2021). *The ultimate guide to implementing wellbeing programmes for school*. Routledge.

Prilleltensky, I., & Prilleltensky, O. (2021). *How people matter: Why it affects health, happiness, love, work, and society*. Cambridge University Press.

Capitalisation

For years, psychologists believed that how couples argue best predicted their happiness and relationship longevity (e.g. Gottman & Silver, 2000). However, they increasingly claim that it is how we respond to each other's good news every day that matters more in the context of enhancing our relationships (Gable et al., 2004). Good news occurs more frequently than arguments; hence we have more opportunities every day of improving our relationships by capitalising. Capitalisation response refers to reacting to other people's good news with genuine interest and enthusiasm (active-constructive), as opposed to ignoring it (passive-destructive), searching for downside to the good news (active-destructive), or half-heartedly (passive-constructive) acknowledging other people's success (Gable & Reis, 2010). Capitalisation is fuelled by positive emotions (Kaczmarek et al., 2021). While we have good evidence showing the positive impact on those who choose to share their news, we also have growing benefits for those who choose to respond in an active-constructive way (Peters et al., 2018). Therefore, the two people involved in a positive exchange gain a lot from it, as they feel closer to their partner and their relationship flourishes (Woods et al., 2015).

Capitalising on good news doesn't come easily to everyone. For example, individuals experiencing social anxiety are less likely to give and receive capitalisation, which leads to the relationship quality declining within as much as 6 months (Kashdan et al., 2013).

Research-based tools

Tool 87: Capitalisation (Lambert et al., 2013)

Write down what went well for you in a diary for 2 weeks and share your personal experiences with your partner at least twice a week.

Variations of practice

While we focused primarily on couples in this section, it is worth noting that you can practise this activity with other family members, friends, neighbours, colleagues at work, and some strangers (when appropriate).

Mental and physical health benefits

Seeking others out and sharing with them the good news is associated with experiences of positive emotions and higher levels of individual and relationship wellbeing than keeping the good news to ourselves (Gable et al., 2004). Furthermore, when partners capitalised on good news, the couple reported higher levels of couple identity, which, over the long term, is also associated with wellbeing (Pagani et al., 2020). Experiencing stress and depression is associated with chronic inflammation, making us less resistant to fighting illness. However, capitalisation buffers this effect, as individuals who practice capitalisation and experience stress and depression are less likely to experience chronic inflammation than those who do not capitalise (Gouin et al., 2020). Furthermore, it is useful when a partner experiences illness. Capitalising predicted daily intimacy between couples when one partner was undergoing cancer treatment (Otto et al., 2015). While more research is required with more diverse groups of people, the existing research suggests ample benefits from this simple process of capitalising.

Caveat

You may be with your partner for a long time, and you are both used to the way you communicate with each other; hence, becoming enthusiastic about their good news may seem out of character for you. Decide the level of enthusiasm with which you want to communicate. It needs to work for you and your partner.

References

Gable, S. L., & Reis, H. T. (2010). Good news! Capitalizing on positive events in an interpersonal context. In M. P. Zanna (Ed.), *Advances in experimental social psychology* (Vol. 42, pp. 195–257). Academic Press. https://doi-org.elib.tcd.ie/10.1016/S0065-2601(10)42004-3

Gable, S. L., Reis, H. T., Impett, E., & Asher, E. R. (2004). What do you do when things go right? The intrapersonal and interpersonal benefits of sharing positive events. *Journal of Personality and Social Psychology, 87*(2), 228–245.

Gottman, J., & Silver, N. (2000). *The seven principles for making marriage work*. Orion Books.

Gouin, J. P., Wrosch, C., McGrath, J., & Booij, L. (2020). Interpersonal capitalization moderates the associations of chronic caregiving stress and depression with inflammation. *Psychoneuroendocrinology*, 112. https://doi-org.elib.tcd.ie/10.1016/j.psyneuen.2019.104509

Kaczmarek, L. D., Kashdan, T. B., Behnke, M., Dziekan, M., Matuła, E., Kosakowski, M., Enko, J., & Guzik, P. (2021). Positive emotions boost enthusiastic responsiveness to capitalization attempts Dissecting self-report, physiology, and behavior. *Journal of Happiness Studies: An Interdisciplinary Forum on Subjective Well-Being*. https://doi-org.elib.tcd.ie/10.1007/s10902-021-00389-y

Kashdan, T. B., Ferssizidis, P., Farmer, A. S., Adams, L. M., & McKnight, P. E. (2013). Failure to capitalize on sharing good news with romantic partners: Exploring positivity deficits of socially anxious people with self-reports, partner-reports, and behavioral observations. *Behaviour Research and Therapy*, *51*(10), 656–668. https://doi.org/10.1016/j.brat.2013.04.006

Lambert, N. M., Gwinn, A. M., Baumeister, R. F., Strachman, A., Washburn, I. J., Gable, S. L., & Fincham, F. D. (2013). A boost of positive affect: The perks of sharing positive experiences. *Journal of Social and Personal Relationships*, *30*(1), 24–43. https://doi-org.elib.tcd.ie/10.1177/0265407512449400

Otto, A. K., Laurenceau, J. P., Siegel, S. D., & Belcher, A. J. (2015). Capitalizing on everyday positive events uniquely predicts daily intimacy and wellbeing in couples coping with breast cancer. *Journal of Family Psychology: JFP: Journal of the Division of Family Psychology of the American Psychological Association* (Division 43), *29*(1), 69–79. https://doi.org/10.1037/fam0000042

Pagani, A. F., Parise, M., Donato, S., Gable, S. L., & Schoebi, D. (2020). If you shared my happiness, you are part of me: Capitalization and the experience of couple identity. *Personality and Social Psychology Bulletin*, *46*(2), 258–269. https://doi.org/10.1177/0146167219854444

Peters, B. J., Reis, H. T., & Gable, S. L. (2018). Making the good even better: A review and theoretical model of interpersonal capitalization (opens in a new window). *Social and Personality Psychology Compass*, 12, e12407.

Woods, S., Lambert, N., Brown, P., Fincham, F., & May, R. (2015). 'I'm so excited for you!' How an enthusiastic responding intervention enhances close relationships. *Journal of Social and Personal Relationships*, *32*(1), 24–40. https://doi-org.elib.tcd.ie/10.1177/0265407514523545

Forgiveness

Forgiveness is one of the most misunderstood concepts in psychology. Often, when people say they do not want to forgive, what they mean is that they condemn what has happened to them and do not want to offer a pardon to the person who did them wrong. However, forgiveness is not about the perpetrator, it is about the self; the perpetrator is irrelevant. You can experience forgiveness at two distinct levels: (1) cognitive, whereby you decide to take steps to forgive, such as completing the tools that follow; and (2) affective, whereby you let go of the experiences of negative emotions. Affective forgiveness is difficult but most beneficial to the self.

It is a process of letting go of the adverse baggage associated with a transgression. Instead of negative, it is about experiencing neutral or positive emotions about the transgressor and the associated situation. Forgiveness takes time, but the activities below may help you speed up this process.

Research-based tools

Tool 88: Letter of forgiveness (adapted from Worthington et al., 2000)

Over the next 30 minutes, write a letter to someone who did you harm. In the letter, (a) describe the event briefly; (b) describe your understanding of the motives of the offender; (c) describe the reasons for wanting to forgive them; and (d) state that you forgive the person who hurt or offended you.

Variations of practice

Instead of the letter of forgiveness, you may choose to practice forgiveness meditation, whereby you meditate on forgiveness and evoke the emotion of forgiveness. In a 2-week community "Forgiveness Blitz" campaign, a range of forgiveness activities was organised for the community to sample, the objective of which was to help them forgive (Brandon et al., 2019). Two activities stood out. The first one was straightforward; it encouraged participants to watch movies about forgiveness and, ideally, have an opportunity to discuss them with someone. Another activity was the Forgiveness Rock Garden, a space in the garden filled with stones with the word "forgive" labelling them. Participants were then asked to perceive a grudge they held against someone as a heavy weight, just like the rocks they were looking at. As soon as they forgave someone for something, they were encouraged to take one rock out of the rock garden to symbolise their act of forgiveness. Finally, there are several therapeutic programmes aimed to help people forgive. One of them is Enright's process model of forgiveness (Enright & Fitzgibbons, 2015), which a therapist usually introduces. Researchers tested it in various populations, such as the elderly, terminally ill cancer patients, women with fibromyalgia, female incest survivors, victims of abuse, and many more (Tsan & Martin, 2021).

Mental and physical health benefits

Forgiving others for their wrongdoings is effective in reducing depression, anger, hostility, stress, and distress, as well as enhancing the experiences of positive emotions (Akhtar & Barlow, 2018). Individuals who were able to forgive reported higher levels of subjective wellbeing (happiness) and greater life satisfaction (Gao et al., 2022). Therefore, forgiveness is beneficial to mental health.

A meta-analysis of studies including more than 58,000 participants showed a relationship between forgiveness and physical health (Lee & Enright, 2019), meaning that those who forgave others have higher levels of physical health. The brain activity of a person who lacks forgiveness is similar to that of those who experience a stressful situation (Worthington, 2006). In contrast, forgiving others results in a range of positive processes in the body, such as lowering blood pressure and heart variation and decreasing physical disease risk by producing low-density lipoproteins (Thoresen et al., 2000). Furthermore, forgiving others significantly improves the immune system and releases antibodies, meaning that you are protected against illness (Worthington & Scherer, 2004). Thus, the research supports the view of forgiveness as a beneficial act to the forgiver's health.

Caveats

Forgiving others is sometimes associated with individuals experiencing mixed emotions. As they write about other people's acts which they choose to forgive, at the same time, they may feel guilty for how they have contributed to the transgressor's behaviour. Also, using this tool may bring many memories of negative and upsetting situations that happened in the past. Please complete it in a safe environment when you have a mental health professional supporting you. Most importantly, however, you should not practise forgiveness in all situations. For example, when partners did not express forgiveness in abusive relationships, the psychological and physical abuse deteriorated over time (McNulty, 2011). At the same time, when abused partners expressed forgiveness, they were less likely to take action to remove themselves from the situation. Also, after expressing forgiveness, they were more likely to return to their abusive partners (Gordon et al., 2004). For self-forgiveness, please go to the self-compassion section of this book.

References

Akhtar, S., & Barlow, J. (2018). Forgiveness therapy for the promotion of mental wellbeing: A systematic review and meta-analysis. *Trauma, Violence, & Abuse, 19*(1), 107–122. https://doi-org.elib.tcd.ie/10.1177/1524838016637079

Enright, R. D., & Fitzgibbons, R. P. (2015). *Forgiveness therapy: An empirical guide to resolving anger and restoring hope.* American Psychological Association.

Gao, F., Li, Y., & Bai, X. (2022). Forgiveness and subjective wellbeing: A meta-analysis review. *Personality & Individual Differences*, *186*, N.PAG. https://doi-org.elib.tcd.ie/10.1016/j.paid.2021.111350

Gordon, N. F., Gulanick, M., Costa, F., Fletcher, G., Franklin, B. A., Roth, E. J., Shephard, T., & American Heart Association Council on Clinical Cardiology, Subcommittee on Exercise, Cardiac Rehabilitation, and Prevention; the Council on Cardiovascular Nursing; the Council on Nutrition, Physical Activity, and Metabolism; and the Stroke Council. (2004). Physical activity and exercise recommendations for stroke survivors: An American Heart Association scientific statement from the Council on Clinical Cardiology, Subcommittee on Exercise, Cardiac Rehabilitation, and Prevention; the Council on Cardiovascular Nursing; the Council on Nutrition, Physical Activity, and Metabolism; and the Stroke Council. *Circulation*, *109*(16), 2031–2041. https://doi.org/10.1161/01.CIR.0000126280.65777.A4

Griffin, B. J., Toussaint, L. L., Zoelzer, M., Worthington Jr., E. L., Coleman, J. A., Lavelock, C. R., McElroy, A., Hook, J. N., Wade, N. G., Sandage, S. J., & Rye, M. S. (2019). Evaluating the effectiveness of a community-based forgiveness campaign. *The Journal of Positive Psychology*, *14*(3), 354–361. doi:10.1080/17439760.2018.1437464

Lee, Y.-R., & Enright, R. D. (2019). A meta-analysis of the association between forgiveness of others and physical health. *Psychology & Health*, *34*(5), 626–643. https://doi-org.elib.tcd.ie/10.1080/08870446.2018.1554185

McNulty, J. K. (2011). The dark side of forgiveness: The tendency to forgive predicts continued psychological and physical aggression in marriage. *Personality and Social Psychology Bulletin*, *37*(6), 770–783. https://doi.org/10.1177/0146167211407077

Thoresen, C. E., Harris, A. H., & Luskin, F. (2000). Forgiveness and health. In M. E. McCullough, K. I. Pargament, & C. E. Thoresen (Eds.), *Forgiveness: Theory, research, and practice* (pp. 254–280). Guilford Press. doi:10.1177/1359105314544132

Tsan, J. A., & Martin, S. R. (2021). Forgiveness. In C. R. Snyder, S. J. Lopez, L. M. Edwards, & S. C. Marques (Eds.), *The Oxford handbook of positive psychology* (pp. 551–570). Oxford University Press.

Worthington, E. L. Jr. (2006). *Forgiveness and reconciliation: Theory and application*. Routledge.

Worthington, E. L. Jr., Kurusu, T. A., Collins, W., Berry, J. W., Ripley, J. S., & Baier, S. N. (2000). Forgiving usually takes time: A lesson learnt by studying interventions to promote forgiveness. *Journal of Psychology and Theology*, *28*(1), 3–20.

Worthington, E. L. Jr., & Scherer, M. (2004). Forgiveness is an emotion-focused coping strategy that can reduce health risks and promote health resilience: Theory, review, and hypotheses. *Psychology and Health*, *19*, 385–405. doi:10.1080/0887044042000196674

Kindness

There have been many calls for us to be kinder to one another in our times. Kindness refers to our actions to benefit others (Curry et al., 2018). It is a fundamental part of humanity to help others. Since pre-historic times, we lived in social groups, and to survive, we helped each other. Therefore, it often comes easily to us, as we have developed this strength for generations, some to a greater extent than others.

We practice various types of kindness:

- Kin altruism means that we are well used to being kind and helpful to our family members, e.g. picking up a child from school or visiting a hospital when someone is sick.
- Mutualism means that we express kindness towards our community, e.g. getting involved in a community cleaning project or coming to help a neighbour when their house was broken into.
- Reciprocal altruism means we are kind to those who may return a favour in the future, e.g. helping an elderly lady cross the road or returning a wallet you found on the street.
- Competitive altruism means that we donate money to charities to improve our status or gain tax credits, or we offer to pay for someone to show them we are wealthier.

Regardless of the type of altruism we practice, the good news is that it can be done anywhere and at any time. As the Dalai Lama famously said on a visit to Capitol Hill in the U.S., "Be kind whenever possible. It is always possible". So let's begin.

Research-based practice

Tool 89: Random acts of kindness (adapted from Curry et al., 2018)

Over the next 7 days, perform at least one act of kindness. A random act of kindness can be any action that is undertaken to be nice to others with no expectation of anything in return. Here are a few examples:

- Holding a door open for a stranger
- Helping shoppers to carry heavy bags
- Paying for the coffee of a random stranger
- Allowing drivers to merge into traffic
- Leaving change in places where it might be helpful
- Commenting positively on a social media message
- Smiling and greeting a person you don't know
- Giving someone a compliment
- Picking up litter and throwing it away

Tool 90: Not-so-random acts of kindness (adapted from Binfet, 2015)

Rather than reacting to the situations you witness and performing your acts of kindness randomly, try to plan for them. In the morning, think of what act of kindness you could perform and who you could be kind to. Then do it.

Tool 91: Counting kindness (adapted from Otake et al., 2006)

Keep track of the kindness you are performing each day for the next 7 days.

Tool 92: Recall acts of kindness (adapted from Ko et al., 2021)

For the next 3 days, take a few minutes to recall an act of kindness you've performed in the past. Try to relive that moment, paying attention to your thoughts and emotions.

Tool 93: Perform or observe (adapted from Rowland & Curry, 2019)

Every day for the next 7 days, observe acts of kindness or perform them.

Tool 94: Pro-social spending (adapted from Dunn et al., 2008)

Over the next week, spend a small amount of money on someone else, such as your family, a friend, or a stranger, or donate money to charity.

Tool 95: Gift of time (adapted from Gander et al., 2013)

Over the next week, meet three of your friends, family members, or colleagues that you care about and offer them your gift of time. Make sure that these are additional activities, not already planned.

Variations of practice

These are just a few ideas. There are unlimited options for showing kindness! For more inspiration, visit the Random Acts of Kindness Foundation (2022). In addition to one-off, spontaneous acts of kindness, why not consider longer-term positive contributions to community projects, charitable foundations, local clubs, or online projects. For example, you could give your time to support vaccination campaigns, offer to read with students at your local school, or even offer accommodation to people who need shelter. Being kind, whether through random acts of kindness or longer-term involvement, will be suitable for the recipients of the kindness whilst also giving your wellbeing a boost. Recently, music making with pre-school children resulted in increased levels of kindness (Beck & Rieser, 2022). This is a very promising activity to teach young children the concept of kindness by experiencing it.

Check out other tools in this book

Self-compassion tools may be beneficial alongside kindness tools.

Mental and physical health benefits

Performing five acts of kindness on a specific day every week for 6 weeks increased participants' levels of happiness (Lyubormirsky et al., 2005). Participants who regularly practiced a variety of random acts of kindness reported increases in happiness during the 10-week period of the research (Sheldon et al., 2013). Therefore, the longer we do it, the longer our increased happiness levels will last. The researchers suggested that when the participants of the study engaged in acts of kindness, it boosted their self-regard and their positive feelings for others and the wider community. Furthermore, kindness resulted in an increase of self-esteem and self-efficacy in students (Datu et al., 2021), whereas not-so-random acts of kindness can also increase perspective, as they allow us to look ahead and plan for kindness (Binfet, 2015). Kindness is particularly beneficial in schools, as it helps students improve mood, affect, and resilience and reduces social interaction anxiety (Shillington et al., 2021). It is also beneficial for reducing symptoms of depression (Mongrain et al., 2018).

In addition to increasing levels of happiness, health and wellbeing benefits have been reported when people are kind to others (Poulin, 2014; Weinstein & Ryan, 2010). It was also one of the activities that reduced pain in adults with chronic illness (Mistretta & Davis, 2021). It was also used as one of many interventions conducted with cancer patients, and it showed reduction in depressive symptoms (Cheung et al., 2017). However, further research is required to identify the impact of performing kindness on other types of physical illness.

Caveats

While being kind is recommended in most situations, the research to date does raise interesting questions. For example, it seems that regularly doing the same act of kindness might reduce the benefits of the positive psychology intervention because it can become mundane

(Lyubormirsky et al., 2005). On the other hand, Sheldon, Boehm, and Lyubormirsky found that intensive periods of random acts of kindness had more positive effects than more less intensive acts of kindness spread out across time (2013). In other words, it may be more beneficial to spend a day volunteering to pick up litter in your neighbourhood than taking on long-term commitments in community projects. Further, some acts of kindness may put you at risk. For example, befriending a homeless person may have some benefits but may also carry an element of risk. So you should be aware of the potential risks of interacting with strangers and take appropriate precautions before engaging in acts of kindness.

References

Beck, S. L., & Rieser, J. (2022). Non-random acts of kindness: Joint music making increases preschoolers' helping and sharing with an adult. *Psychology of Music*, *50*(1), 17–33. https://doi-org.elib.tcd.ie/10.1177/0305735620978688

Binfet, J.-T. (2015). Not-so random acts of kindness: A guide to intentional kindness in the classroom. *The International Journal of Emotional Education*, *7*(2), 49–62.

Cheung, E. O., Cohn, M. A., Dunn, L. B., Melisko, M. E., Morgan, S., Penedo, F. J., Salsman, J. M., Shumay, D. M., & Moskowitz, J. T. (2017). A randomized pilot trial of a positive affect skill intervention (lessons in linking affect and coping) for women with metastatic breast cancer. *Psycho-Oncology*, *26*(12), 2101–2108. https://doi-org.elib.tcd.ie/10.1002/pon.4312

Curry, O. S., Rowland, L. A., Van Lissa, C. J., Zlotowitz, S., McAlaney, J., & Whitehouse, H. (2018). Happy to help? A systematic review and meta-analysis of the effects of performing acts of kindness on the wellbeing of the actor. *Journal of Experimental Social Psychology*, *76*, 320–329.

Datu, J. A. D., Ping Wong, G. S., & Rubie-Davies, C. (2021). Can kindness promote media literacy skills, self-esteem, and social self-efficacy among selected female secondary school students? An intervention study. *Computers & Education*, *161*. https://doi-org.elib.tcd.ie/10.1016/j.compedu.2020.104062

Dunn, E. W., Aknin, L. B., & Norton, M. I. (2008). Spending money on others promotes happiness. *Science (New York, N.Y.)*, *319*(5870), 1687–1688. https://doi.org/10.1126/science.1150952

Gander, F., Proyer, R., Ruch, W., & Wyss, T. (2013). Strength-based positive interventions: Further evidence for their potential in enhancing well-being and alleviating depression. *Journal of Happiness Studies*, *14*(4), 1241–1259.

Ko, Kellon, Margolis, Seth, Revord, Julia, & Lyubomirsky, Sonja. (2021). Comparing the effects of performing and recalling acts of kindness. *The Journal of Positive Psychology*, *16*(1), 73–81. doi:10.1080/17439760.2019.1663252

Lyubormirsky, S., Sheldon, K. M., & Schkade, D. (2005). Pursuing happiness: The architecture of sustainable change. *Review of General Psychology*, *9*, 111–131.

Mistretta, E. G., & Davis, M. C. (2021). Meta-analysis of self-compassion interventions for pain and psychological symptoms among adults with chronic illness. *Mindfulness*. https://doi-org.elib.tcd.ie/10.1007/s12671-021-01766-7

Mongrain, M., Barnes, C., Barnhart, R., & Zalan, L. B. (2018). Acts of kindness reduce depression in individuals low on agreeableness. *Translational Issues in Psychological Science*, *4*(3), 323–334. https://doi.org/10.1037/tps0000168

Poulin, M. J. (2014). Volunteering predicts health among those who value others: Two national studies. *Health Psychology*, *33*(2), 120–129.

Random Acts of Kindness Foundation. Retrieved January 8, 2022, from randomactsofkindness.org

Rowland, L., & Curry, O. S. (2019). A range of kindness activities boost happiness. *The Journal of Social Psychology*, *159*(3), 340–343.

Sheldon, K. M., Boehm, J., & Lyubormirsky, S. (2013). Variety is the spice of happiness. The hedonic adaptation prevention model. In S. A. David, I. Boniwell, & A. C. Ayers (Eds.), *The Oxford handbook of happiness* (pp. 901–914). Oxford University Press.

Shillington, K. J., Johnson, A. M., Mantler, T., Burke, S. M., & Irwin, J. D. (2021). Kindness as an intervention for student social interaction anxiety, resilience, affect, and mood: The kiss of kindness study ii. *Journal of Happiness Studies: An Interdisciplinary Forum on Subjective Well-Being*. https://doi-org.elib.tcd.ie/10.1007/s10902-021-00379-0

Weinstein, N., & Ryan, R. M. (2010). When helping helps: Autonomous motivation for prosocial behavior and its influence on well-being for the helper and recipient. *Journal of Personality and Social Psychology*, *98*(2), 222–244.

Savouring relationships

Savouring is an act of directing our attention to, taking steps to improve, and appreciating positive experiences in our lives (Bryant & Veroff, 2007). We can savour events in the past (see the Reminiscence tools), present (see the Meditation tools), or the future (see the Appreciation tools). The skill of savouring requires us to direct our attention to the specific details of an object or event and engage our senses to be present in the experience fully. Since it involves paying attention to detail, it often involves slowing down to give the experience our full attention. In addition, it is extended beyond our sensory experience to include our capacity to reflect on experience using our thought processes. There are ten strategies for experiencing savouring, according to Bryant and Veroff (2007). In what follows, you will find examples that focus on using these strategies for savouring relationships in particular.

1 Sharing positive experiences with others, e.g. boost your bonding with your family and friends by doing something enjoyable together.
2 Memory building, e.g. as you are having a great time with others, now and then, stop and take a "mental photograph" of this moment to help you re-experience it later.
3 Comparing, e.g. reflect on how lucky you are with your relationships with your partner, child, and friends and think of why when comparing it with other people.

4 Sensory perceptual sharpening, e.g. as you are having dinner with your partner, focus on specific stimuli, be it the touch of a hand or their sparkling eyes, while consciously blocking other parts.
5 Self-congratulations, e.g. congratulate yourself on the relationships you've developed to date; tell yourself how proud you are of what you created together with a person or people. This could be settling into a new role at work or overcoming a conflict with your friend.
6 Absorption, e.g. when playing with your children, get into a state of flow in which you lose yourself entirely in the activity you're performing.
7 Behavioural expression, e.g. dance, sing, laugh, giggle, smile together.
8 Temporal awareness, e.g. acknowledge the fleeting moments in your life, how an event you have been waiting for has come and fast it is coming to an end, or how fast your children grow. Consciously enjoy every moment of it.
9 Count blessings, e.g. remind yourself of your good fortune, be thankful for the people in your life and your relationship with them.
10 Killjoy thinking (reverse), e.g. when you are experiencing a great time with someone or your relationship with someone is going well, stop worrying and ruminating about it not lasting (killjoy thinking). Just enjoy the good relationship you have now.

Those were some of the generic recommendations on how to experience savouring. In this section, you will also find research-based tools for doing it.

Research-based tools

Tool 96: Remembering past events (Biskas et al., 2019)

Bring to mind a positive event involving other people from the past, e.g. friendships in school, meeting your partner, getting married. Immerse yourself in the memories you have by thinking about the situation associated with your memory and how it made you feel. Write down four key words that best describe your memories and then spend 5 to 10 minutes writing down the details of your experience and how it made you feel.

Tool 97: Relationship savouring for young people (Borelli et al., 2020)

Think of someone in your life to whom you turn for support and comfort. Reflect on a specific time in the past when:

> That person gave you loving care when you needed it, e.g. when you were upset or feeling lonely.

That person supported you in taking a risk you would not have otherwise taken.

That person offered you closeness that allowed you to feel safe, loved, connected, and appreciated.

Tool 98: Savouring your child (adapted from Burkhart et al., 2015, p. 699)

Sit down and think about an experience with your child which evoked positive emotions with you. It can be as simple as taking their hand while walking to school, going to a park, or holidays. Focus on a specific memory when you connect with your child. Think or write down in detail what happened: What were the circumstances? What was the weather like? What were you both wearing? What have you seen around you? What were you thinking? What were you feeling? Now, reflect on your thoughts and feelings about your relationship with your child.

Tool 99: Shared connection (adapted from Zhou et al., 2022)

Watch the following video: www.youtube.com/watch?v=fHoEWUTYnSo, which shows Barbara Fredrickson discussing the concept of positivity resonance. Set a phone reminder in the morning that will remind you to experience more social connections every day for the next 7 days, e.g. a mutual smile, a laugh, an act of kindness with strangers (if safe), acquaintances, colleagues, friends, or family members. In the evening, reflect on how each connection made a difference in your life today.

Variations of practice

When you're embarking on a new relationship, you can use some savouring activities to help you first anticipate and savour the present and then move towards thinking of memories you've created. These activities are for all stages of relationships.

Mental and physical health benefits

Practising savouring is associated with both an increase in positive emotion (Wilson & MacNamara, 2021) and a decrease in negative emotion (Bryant & Veroff, 2007). Practising savouring contributes to hedonic happiness or the feeling that we are living a pleasant life (Bryant & Veroff, 2007). In a relational context, it is associated with relationship satisfaction between life partners Lenger & Gordon, 2019).

Furthermore, anticipation savouring in couples (thinking about positive experiences in the future) is correlated with relationship satisfaction. In contrast, couples savoured the present moment; they were more likely to report subjective wellbeing (Singh & Tripathi, 2018). Savouring is particularly good for acting as a buffer when couples experience stressful times, allowing them to pull together instead of pulling apart (Samios & Khatri, 2019).

Concerning children–parent relationships, the savouring moments adults experience with their children boost their positive affect and improve their relationship (Burkhart et al., 2015). Savouring was particularly useful for parents of toddlers, as it improves their emotional state (having young children is often associated with sleep debt and increase of negative emotions due to daily hassles) and created greater closeness between toddlers and parents, if parents tended to display avoidant attachment style, for at least 2 years after the intervention (Burkhart et al., 2015). However, this effect is relevant mainly for relational savouring (e.g. savouring a relationship you have with your child); thus, if you choose to do personal savouring (e.g. savouring a quiet cup of tea), your positive experience will still be there. Still, its impact on your relationship satisfaction may remain the same. Finally, a savouring tool was introduced to teens in a residential facility (Wang et al., 2019). Many of them had unhelpful attitudes and beliefs towards relationships, and the activity helped them improve their beliefs. Thus, relationship savouring can be particularly valuable for those who have previously experienced unhealthy relationships.

In relation to physical health, savouring moderates the correlation between cancer-specific symptoms and depression (Hou et al., 2017); thus, it helps when individuals are going through difficult times in their lives. This was also the case for some of the partners of cancer patients, who often experience higher levels of distress during their intimate partner's therapy (Holness, 2018). Post-chemotherapy, when practising relational savouring, those securely attached benefited from the activity, whereas those who experienced relational anxiety and avoidance found this activity more upsetting. When savouring was introduced to a group of elderly, their cardiovascular health improved following the intervention (Borelli et al., 2019).

Caveat

Savouring may have a limited impact on people who already experience positive relationships. Research shows that the most significant impact on parent–child relationships is in parents who have avoidant attachment and may benefit from reducing negative emotions that the savouring exercise brings. Savouring exercises are complex in that they have been found to both reduce negative emotions and increase positive emotions. This suggests that while there is a positive impact even on people who are not in distress, the impact of savouring will be most keenly felt when one needs emotional regulation (reduction in negative emotions).

References

Biskas, M., Cheung, W. Y., Juhl, J., Sedikides, C., Wildschut, T., & Hepper, E. (2019). A prologue to nostalgia: Savouring creates nostalgic memories that foster optimism. *Cognition & Emotion*, *33*(3), 417–427. https://doi.org/10.1080/02699 931.2018.1458705

Borelli, J. L., Bond, D. K., Fox, M., & Horn Mallers, M. (2019). Relational savoring reduces physiological reactivity and enhances psychological agency of older adults. *Journal of Applied Gerontology*. doi:10.1177/0733464819866972

Borelli, J. L., Smiley, P. A., Kerr, M. L., Hong, K., Hecht, H. K., Blackard, M. B., Falasiri, E., Cervantes, B. R., & Bond, D. K. (2020). Relational savoring: An attachment-based approach to promoting interpersonal flourishing. *Psychotherapy*, *57*(3), 340–351. https://doi.org/10.1037/pst0000284

Bryant, F. B., & Veroff, J. (2007). *Savoring: A new model of positive experience*. Taylor Francis Group.

Burkhart, M. L., Borelli, J. L., Rasmussen, H. F., & Sbarra, D. A. (2015). Cherish the good times: Relational savoring in parents of infants and toddlers. *Personal Relationships*, *22*(4), 692–711. https://doi-org.elib.tcd.ie/10.1111/pere.12104

Holness, A. E. (2018). Relational savoring among intimate partners of cancer patients [ProQuest Information & Learning]. *Dissertation Abstracts International: Section B: The Sciences and Engineering*, *79*(4–B(E)).

Hou, W. K., Lau, K. M., Ng, S. M., Cheng, A. C. K., Shum, T. C. Y., Cheng, S., & Cheung, H. Y. S. (2017). Savoring moderates the association between cancer-specific physical symptoms and depressive symptoms. *Psycho-Oncology*, *26*(2), 231–238. https://doi-org.elib.tcd.ie/10.1002/pon.4114

Lenger, K. A., & Gordon, C. L. (2019). To have and to savor: Examining the associations between savoring and relationship satisfaction. *Couple and Family Psychology: Research and Practice*, *8*(1), 1–9. https://doi.org/10.1037/cfp0000111

Samios, C., & Khatri, V. (2019). When times get tough: Savoring and relationship satisfaction in couples coping with a stressful life event. *Anxiety, Stress & Coping: An International Journal*, *32*(2), 125–140.

Singh, U., & Tripathi, A. (2018). Savoring beliefs, relationship satisfaction and subjective wellbeing among married couples. *International Journal of Movement Education and Social Science*, *7*(1), 315–323.

Wang, B. A., Bouche, V., Hong, K., Eriksen, D. E., Rice, R., & Borelli, J. L. (2021). Investigating the efficacy of relational savoring among male adolescents in residential treatment. *Residential Treatment for Children & Youth*, *38*(3), 307–323. https://doi-org.elib.tcd.ie/10.1080/0886571X.2019.1707146

Wilson, K. A., & MacNamara, A. (2021). Savor the moment: Willful increase in positive emotion and the persistence of this effect across time. *Psychophysiology, 58*(3), e13754–n/a. https://doi.org/10.1111/psyp.13754

Zhou, J., Prinzing, M. M., Le Nguyen, K. D., West, T. N., & Fredrickson, B. L. (2022). The goods in everyday love: Positivity resonance builds prosociality. *Emotion, 22*(1), 30–45. https://doi.org/10.1037/emo0001035

Your reflection space

Which relationship tools would you like to try? Why?
Which activities did you find most useful? How did you tweak them?

8 Prospecting

Prospecting is about a future focus (Seligman et al., 2016). For many people, the future is filled with possibilities. Young people look forward to getting older and finally being able to take ownership of their lives, moving out of their family home, travelling the world, and having the time of their lives. Young adults look forward to developing their dream career, getting married, buying their first home, and having a family. We all look forward to bigger and smaller events in our lives, such as holidays, weddings, and meeting friends. Thinking about them fills us up with a burst of positive emotions. They have the power of transforming even the most challenging day into a hopeful moment. This is the power of our imagination.

In the same way, as we can see our future as hopeful, it can also affect us negatively. Three types of "faulty" prospections may contribute significantly to developing depression (Roepke & Seligman, 2016):

1 Negative beliefs about the future relate to our attitudes and beliefs about the world around us, not necessarily relating to our lives, e.g. the future is a brewing disaster, politically and economically.
2 Poor generation of potential in the future relates to having many negative scenarios floating in our heads about our lives and what we can accomplish, e.g. unless I get this job, my life will continue to go nowhere.
3 Poor evaluation of what the future may bring relates to having negative expectations and predictions of the future, e.g. no matter if I get this job or not, life will be just as bad as it is now.

This section will discuss the tools that may help you change your future into a more positive one and hopefully result in higher wellbeing.

The prospecting tools include:

1. Anticipation
2. Goal setting
3. Best possible self
4. Hope

References

Roepke, A. M., & Seligman, M. E. P. (2016). Depression and prospection. *British Journal of Clinical Psychology*, 55(1), 23–48. https://doi-org.elib.tcd.ie/10.1111/bjc.12087

Seligman, M. E. P., Railton, P., Baumeister, R. F., & Sripada, C. (2016). *Homo prospectus*. Oxford University Press.

Anticipation

The work of Sigmund Freud has influenced millions of people worldwide. Subsequently, therapists and psychologists began to focus on how their clients' past events got in the way of thriving today. In contrast, we discussed little about the future and how the future influenced our actions today. Yet we are *homo prospectus*, not only *homo sapiens* (Seligman et al., 2016); as such, we are oriented towards the future, with our ultimate goal being survival. The reason we don't want to do something today might not be because we had a toxic childhood or underwent other adverse life experiences but because we are anxious about the future, anxious about the consequences of today's actions tomorrow.

Similarly, focusing our attention on the future can offer us comfort and become a source of psychological flourishing. This is partially the role that anticipation plays in our lives. Anticipation is a component of savouring (Bryant, 2003). It refers to looking forward to the positive events in our lives, feeling joy about anticipating the future, daydreaming about the future positive events, and imagining the consequences of the future when all has gone well for us.

The ability to anticipate is a privilege. Animals are incapable of it; hence it is a special gift bestowed upon us due to our prefrontal cortex developing to the extent it has. We know this because patients with damage to this part of the brain cannot do it (Melges, 1990). This is why we should use this gift as much as possible, especially since we know it can boost our wellbeing. What is also going well for us is that we usually tend to overestimate how much happier we will be after the positive event (Gilbert & Wilson, 2007). This is why anticipation can help us get the best out of our lives today and tomorrow.

Research-based tools

Tool 100: Looking forward to tomorrow (adapted from Littman-Ovadia & Nir, 2014)

Every day, over the next 7 days, take 5 minutes to write down three good things (people or events) that you are looking forward to experiencing tomorrow. Then, select one thing that you are waiting for, and for the next 5 minutes, try to experience it wholeheartedly ahead of time.

Tool 101: Positive mental time travel (adapted from Quoidbach et al., 2009)

For the next week, before going to bed, try to vividly imagine four positive events that could happen to you the next day. They can be as simple as getting a text from someone you like, eating your favourite food, or doing your favourite work. Try to use all your senses when imagining the events: sense of smell, touch, sight, etc.

Tool 102: Prospective writing (adapted from Roepke et al., 2018)

If you have recently experienced adversity, carve out 15 minutes of your time once a week for a month to write about your experiences. So many people in these situations feel a sense of loss and realise that some "doors" have now closed and new "doors" have opened or will open. The new opportunities can include engaging in something new, setting up new goals, making new friends, or making life changes. All these new opportunities can exist alongside the losses, and they do not make the losses less painful or unimportant. So please write about the new doors that have opened for you or may open for you in the forthcoming months (future opportunities).

Tool 103: Savouring a film (Chun et al., 2017)

After selecting a film and before watching it, take half a minute or a minute to savour your upcoming movie. You can do it in the cinema or at home. To amplify the joy you will experience from it, continue to savour the film as you are watching it.

Variations of practice

You can use this technique to anticipate any positive events in your lives, be it your upcoming birthday, holidays, meeting with friends, or the weekend. Also, there is another concept related to savouring and anticipating: life longings. Life longings are desires that we all have about our potential future or the past (Scheibe et al., 2007) – the things that we want to happen but we cannot find a way of making happen. For example, childless women may desire to have children. In the absence of children, they imagine the potential life they could have, the joys and challenges of being a mother. While many women may become upset due to this daydreaming, it is a positive experience for some as long as they have control over their dreams and know when to stop (Kotter-Grühn et al., 2009).

Check out other tools in this book

Any Hope tools tap into the power of anticipation. Also, please review the Reminiscing tool and the Savouring Tool, as both reminiscence and anticipation are an integral part of savouring.

Mental and physical wellbeing benefits

Anticipation plays an important evolutionary role, whereby it helps us prepare our strategies (emotional, cognitive, and behavioural) to cope with future events (Gilbert & Wilson, 2007). For example, future focus is associated with school achievement (Vecchio et al., 2021) and can protect young people against risky sexual behaviours, such as not using condoms (Abousselam et al., 2016). Anticipating positive future events, such as holidays, can boost our positive emotions, although, like many emotions, this boost is temporary, and our mindset returns to baseline after the holidays (Nawijn et al., 2010). Reflecting for a week on what we look forward to the next day is associated not only with a temporary boost but also with sustained changes a month later, such as reduced pessimism and emotional exhaustion and improvement of optimistic thinking and positive emotions (Littman-Ovadia & Nir, 2014). Writing about the traumatic event and the future doors it may open resulted in non-clinical participants experiencing higher levels of wellbeing and growth after trauma (Roepke et al., 2018). Thus, thinking about the future working out well can help you greatly enhance positive emotions and develop.

Anticipation is adequate for clinical patients too. Neurological research showed that the lack of anticipation was associated with anxiety and depression (Abler et al., 2007; Heitmann et al., 2014). In patients with schizophrenia, imagining future events improved their clinical symptoms, positive emotions, and life satisfaction Chen et al., 2020). Also, discounting the future thinking is associated with many unhealthy behaviours, as we do not consider the consequences of our actions; however, episodic future thinking (briefly moving into the future to consider the consequences) helps us make better decisions about our health today. This is why the anticipation activity is helpful for anyone who wishes to engage in pro-health behaviour, e.g. quitting smoking, as it is affecting your health very significantly (Hollis-Hansen et al., 2019).

Warning

When engaging in anticipation, we can focus on the potentially positive or negative outcomes. While focusing on the positive outcome can enhance positive emotions, beware that anticipating stress in the morning (not at night) may decline cognition and working memory that day (Hyun et al., 2019). That said, if anticipation is followed up with strategies to overcome adversity, it prepares us to cope with challenges more effectively. Also, sometimes, anticipating positive outcomes and fantasizing about them can backfire, because we are less likely to put effort into the goals we set up. For example, in a study with people who tried to lose weight, those who fantasized about successfully lost weight were successful in accomplishing their endeavour (Oettingen & Wadden, 1991). So, when engaging in this activity, you need to be clear about your aim. Positive anticipation is excellent for improving our emotional wellbeing, but it might not serve us in all life situations.

References

Abler, B., Erk, S., Herwig, U., & Walter, H. (2007). Anticipation of aversive stimuli activates extended amygdala in unipolar depression. *Journal of Psychiatric Research*, *41*(6), 511–522. https://doi-org.elib.tcd.ie/10.1016/j.jpsychires.2006.07.020

Abousselam, N., Naudé, L., Lens, W., & Esterhuyse, K. (2016). The relationship between future time perspective, self-efficacy and risky sexual behaviour in the Black youth of central South Africa. *Journal of Mental Health*, *25*(2), 176–183. https://doi-org.elib.tcd.ie/10.3109/09638237.2015.1078884

Bryant, F. B. (2003). Savoring beliefs inventory (SBI): A scale for measuring beliefs about savouring. *Journal of Mental Health*, *12*(2), 175–196. https://doi.org/10.1080/0963823031000103489

Chen, G., Luo, H., Wu, G., Zhou, C., Wang, K., Feng, K., Xiao, Z., Huang, J., Gan, J., Zhao, P., Liu, P.-Z., & Wang, Y. (2020). Improving mental time travel in schizophrenia: Do remembering the past and imagining the future make a difference? *Cognitive Therapy & Research*, *44*(5), 893–905. https://doi-org.elib.tcd.ie/10.1007/s10608-020-10083-7

Chun, H. H., Diehl, K., & MacInnis, D. J. (2017). Savoring an upcoming experience affects ongoing and remembered consumption enjoyment. *Journal of Marketing*, *81*(3), 96–110. https://doi-org.elib.tcd.ie/10.1509/jm.15.0267

Gilbert, D. T., & Wilson, T. D. (2007). Prospection: Experiencing the future. *Science*, *317*(5843), 1351–1354. https://doi-org.elib.tcd.ie/10.1126/science.1144161

Heitmann, C. Y., Peterburs, J., Mothes, L. M., Hallfarth, M. C., Böhme, S., Miltner, W. H. R., & Straube, T. (2014). Neural correlates of anticipation and processing of performance feedback in social anxiety. *Human Brain Mapping*, *35*(12), 6023–6031. https://doi-org.elib.tcd.ie/10.1002/hbm.22602

Hollis-Hansen, K., O'Donnell, D. S. E., Seidman, J. S., Brande, S. J., & Epstein, L. H. (2019). Improvements in episodic future thinking methodology: Establishing a standardized episodic thinking control. *PLoS One*, *14*(3), 1–13. https://doi-org.elib.tcd.ie/10.1371/journal.pone.0214397

Hyun, J., Sliwinski, M. J., & Smyth, J. M. (2019). Waking up on the wrong side of the bed: The effects of stress anticipation on working memory in daily life. *The Journals of Gerontology. Series B, Psychological Sciences and Social Sciences*, *74*(1), 38–46. https://doi.org/10.1093/geronb/gby042

Kotter-Grühn, D., Scheibe, S., Blanchard-Fields, F., & Baltes, P. B. (2009). Developmental emergence and functionality of Sehnsucht (life longings): The sample case of involuntary childlessness in middle-aged women. *Psychology and Aging*, *24*(3), 634–644. https://doi.org/10.1037/a0016359

Littman-Ovadia, H., & Nir, D. (2014). Looking forward to tomorrow: The buffering effect of a daily optimism intervention. *The Journal of Positive Psychology*, *9*(2), 122–136. https://doi.org/10.1080/17439760.2013.853202

Melges, F. T. (1990). Identity and temporal perspective. In R. A. Block (Ed.), *Cognitive models of psychological time* (pp. 255–266). Erlbaum.

Nawijn, J., Marchand, M. A., Veenhoven, R., & Vingerhoets, A. J. (2010). Vacationers happier, but most not happier after a holiday. *Applied Research in Quality of Life*, *5*(1), 35–47. https://doi-org.elib.tcd.ie/10.1007/s11482-009-9091-9

Oettingen, G., & Wadden, T. A. (1991). Expectation, fantasy, and weight loss: Is the impact of positive thinking always positive? *Cognitive Therapy and Research*, *15*(2), 167–175. https://doi.org/10.1007/BF01173206

Quoidbach, J., Wood, A. M., & Hansenne, M. (2009). Back to the future: The effect of daily practice of mental time travel into the future on happiness and anxiety. *The Journal of Positive Psychology*, *4*(5), 349–355. https://doi-org.elib.tcd.ie/10.1080/17439760902992365

Roepke, Ann Marie, Benson, Lizbeth, Tsukayama, Eli, & Yaden, David Bryce. (2018). Prospective writing: Randomized controlled trial of an intervention for facilitating growth after adversity. *The Journal of Positive Psychology*, *13*(6), 627–642. doi:10.1080/17439760.2017.1365161

Scheibe, S., Freund, A. M., & Baltes, P. B. (2007). Toward a developmental psychology of Sehnsucht (life longings): The optimal (utopian) life. *Developmental Psychology*, *43*(3), 778–795. https://doi.org/10.1037/0012-1649.43.3.778

Seligman, M. E. P., Railton, P., Baumeister, R. F., & Sripada, C. (2016). *Homo prospectus*. Oxford University Press.

Vecchio, G. M., Lonigro, A., Laghi, F., Barcaccia, B., & Pallini, S. (2021). The influence of study interests on school achievement: The role of future time perspective and positive affect. *International Journal of School & Educational Psychology*, *9*, S47–S57. https://doi-org.elib.tcd.ie/10.1080/21683603.2020.1721386

Goal setting

We all do goal setting every day, whether we are aware of it or not. The good news is that the process of setting and achieving goals can be beneficial for your wellbeing (Grant & Spence, 2010). Accomplishing things is a crucial element of wellbeing (Seligman, 2011). This means that being thoughtful about the goals we set for ourselves and then achieving them can be part of our wellbeing strategies.

Research-based practice

Tool 104: Letter from the future (adapted from Hoffman et al., 2010)

Write a letter from your future self to the present self in which you describe all your important goals and ways in which you managed to achieve them to help you live the life you always wanted to live.

The practice is simply to set yourself an achievable goal and then pursue it until you have accomplished it. To gain the most benefits to your wellbeing, ensure that:

- The goal is challenging (not too easy and not impossible)
- The goal is self-selected (something that you have chosen to do)
- The goal is personally meaningful (something that you would be proud to achieve)
- You will be able to determine when it has been achieved
- You can monitor your progress towards the goal.

When you achieve your goal, make sure to find a way to celebrate your success. Doing this will provide you with a wellbeing boost, and it also gives you evidence of your ability to set and achieve tasks.

Variations of practice

Letters from the future come in various forms. You can write a letter to the future self in 20 years from now (Rutchick et al., 2018), or on your specific birthday in the future (Round & Burke, 2018); alternatively, if you are going through a difficult time that is likely to end the following year, you may write a letter from the future self this time next year (Chishima et al., 2021). In some cases, setting ourselves goals that are personally meaningful and simply pursuing them can be good for our wellbeing (Boniwell & Tunariu, 2019). So it may be helpful to set yourself a longer-term goal that resonates with your values and who you are.

The process of working towards an important, meaningful goal is in itself rewarding.

Check out other tools in this book

In the final chapter of this book, we guide you through a goal-setting process.

Mental and physical health benefits

Researchers worldwide have shown that pursuing specific life goals can lead to physical and mental wellbeing (Schmuck & Sheldon, 2001). According to Locke and Latham (2002), setting goals leads to four outcomes:

1 Setting a goal directs our attention. In other words, we are less prone to get distracted.
2 Having a goal can be energising. This is particularly true when we perceive the goal as challenging.
3 A goal can increase our persistence, especially when the goal is self-selected.
4 Working towards a goal leads us to discover the knowledge and skills required to achieve it.

The self-concordance model (Sheldon & Elliott, 1999) suggests that when your goals are consistent (or concordant) with your values and interests, you are more likely to invest more effort towards achieving the goals, thus increasing the likelihood of achieving them. Furthermore, when these self-concordant goals are attained, you are more likely to experience increased wellbeing (Sheldon & Elliott, 1999). In another study, people were supported to develop goal-setting and planning skills. The research showed significant increases in wellbeing, showing that goal-setting and planning skills can lead directly to increases in wellbeing (MacLeod et al., 2008).

Caveat

While setting and achieving goals generally boosts wellbeing, it is essential to note that a study suggests that some people who linked their happiness to the achievement of academic, social, and fitness goals were more at risk of becoming depressed than those who pursued the same goals for enjoyment (Street, 1994). In other words, you should be careful not to think that you will *only* experience wellbeing if and when you achieve your goals. According to the study, making your wellbeing conditional on achieving specific goals can lead to rumination, and that can lead to depression in some instances.

References

Boniwell, I., & Tunariu, A. (2019). *Positive psychology: Theory, research and applications* (2nd ed.). Open University Press.

Chishima, Y., Huai-Ching Liu, I. T., & Wilson, A. E. (2021). Temporal distancing during the COVID-19 pandemic: Letter writing with future self can mitigate negative affect. *Applied Psychology: Health and Well-Being, 13*(2), 406–418. https://doi.org/10.1111/aphw.12256

Grant, A. M., & Spence, G. B. (2010). Using coaching and positive psychology to promote a flourishing workforce: A model of goal-striving and mental health. In P. A. Linley, S. Harrington, & N. Page (Eds.), *Oxford handbook for positive psychology and work* (pp. 175–188). Oxford University Press.

Locke, E. A., & Latham, G. P. (2002). Building a practically useful theory of goal setting and task motivation. *American Psychologist, 57*(9), 705–717.

MacLeod, A. K., Coates, E., & Hetherton, J. (2008). Increasing wellbeing through teaching goal-setting and planning skills: Results of a brief intervention. *Journal of Happiness Studies: An Interdisciplinary Forum on Subjective Well-Being, 9*(2), 185–196.

Round, J., & Burke, J. (2018). A dream of a retirement: The longitudinal experiences and perceived retirement wellbeing of recent retirees following a tailored intervention linking best possible self-expressive writing with goal-setting. *International Coaching Psychology Review, 13*(2), 27–45.

Rutchick, A. M., Slepian, M. L., Reyes, M. O., Pleskus, L. N., & Hershfield, H. E. (2018). Future self-continuity is associated with improved health and increases exercise behavior. *Journal of Experimental Psychology: Applied, 24*(1), 72–80. https://doi.org/10.1037/xap0000153

Schmuck, P., & Sheldon, K. M. (Eds.). (2001). *Life goals and wellbeing: Towards a positive psychology of human striving.* Hogrefe & Huber.

Seligman, M. E. P. (2011). *Flourish: A new understanding of happiness and well-being – and how to achieve them.* Nicholas Brealey.

Sheldon, K. M, & Elliott, A. J. (1999). Goal striving, need satisfaction, and longitudinal wellbeing: The self-concordance model. *Journal of Personality and Social Psychology, 76*, 482–497.

Street, H. (1994). Depression and the pursuit of happiness: An investigation into the relationship between goal setting, goal pursuit and vulnerability to depression. *Clinical Psychologist, 4*, 18–25.

Best possible self

The best possible self is a personal creative writing activity focused on representing our personal goals and dreams about who we want to be in a concrete way (Markus & Nurius, 1986). It focuses on your wishes for yourself and reflects priorities and motivations. The exercise is beneficial because it increases positive emotions. It may also help clarify goals and priorities as we write about our feelings and motivations (Sheldon & Lyubomirsky, 2006). Recently, researchers compared writing about the best possible self in the past, present, and future (Carrillo et al., 2021). Their results showed that changing the temporal perspective can have the same positive effect on your wellbeing.

Research-based tools

Tool 105: Best possible self in the future (adapted from King, 2001)

Take 15 to 20 minutes to sit down and write about yourself in the future. Consider what the future would be like if everything has worked out exactly as you hope it would if you made all your dreams and aspirations come true. Write your experience in detail.

Tool 106: Best possible self in the past (adapted from Carrillo et al., 2021)

Now consider your best past self. Visualise yourself in the past when you were experiencing the best time and considered it the best version of yourself. Write about it in as much detail as you can. Now, refocus your attention on the future and how you can use what you have learnt about your best possible self from the past in the future.

Tool 107: Best possible health (used with permission by Gibson et al., 2021)

"Take a moment to think about your best possible self. Imagine that you are in excellent health and have been taking extra good care of your body. You are exercising regularly, and you are eating well. You have worked hard and succeeded at accomplishing all of your health-related goals. Imagine how it felt to achieve those goals and reflect on how positive it would feel to be this fit and healthy. Then, tell yourself the essential things you realised or the critical steps you took to get there. Now, please use the next 10 minutes to write continuously about what you imagined. Use the tips below to guide you through this process:

1   Be as creative and imaginative as you want. Do not worry about perfect grammar and spelling, as this is for your private use. No one

has to know what you wrote down, though you may find it helpful to share and develop ideas with trusted friends, family, or your healthcare team.
2   Do not feel too pressured to write everything down on your first try. As you repeat this task, more ideas will come to you naturally.
3   Remember, steps towards success are often small. You may find it easier to write about more possible things, to begin with, such as investing in a pedometer/walking app or making the decision to try new recipes more often. However, if you want to aim high and write about running a half-marathon, that's okay too!
4   If you find thinking about one aspect of your health particularly difficult, try focusing on another one. The important thing is that you write about something long term so that you can make more noticeable improvements over time" (Gibson et al., 2021, p. 1716).

Variations of practice

Reflective writing has several benefits. Early research on the benefits of writing focused on writing about traumatic events. It is thought that writing about traumatic events may have a cathartic element. Still, many people do not want to experience negative emotions with this activity. Interestingly, King's work on the best possible self suggests that we can have similar benefits without the burden of recalling past adverse events. The Best Possible Self exercise varies from traditional reflective writing in that it allows the writer to focus on positive experiences (King, 2001).

Mental and physical health benefits

This exercise reduces negative emotion and improves positive emotion (Sheldon & Lyubomirsky, 2006). It is argued that it can help you minimize conflict around your goals by clarifying priorities and supporting motivation (Emmons, 1986; Omodei & Wearing, 1990). Importantly, it has been shown to help with psychological adjustment (Rivkin & Taylor, 1999) by assisting people in integrating their life experiences and giving the writer a greater sense of control over their life (Lyubomirsky et al., 2005). Usually, the activity is carried out with younger people. However, Round and Burke (2018) carried out experimental qualitative research with retirees showing that it can prove effective for enhancing wellbeing and planning for the future.

Concerning physical health, engaging in disclosive writing that asks us to deeply reflect on our thoughts and feelings has been demonstrated to have health benefits. King (2001) showed that participants who wrote about their best possible self experienced less ill health as measured by the number of visits to the health centre. Several other studies on disclosive writing have found health benefits (Cameron & Nicholls, 1998; King & Miner, 2000). It is thought that the benefits come from the increased insight and self-regulation of emotions that the reflection part of the writing enables (King, 2001).

Caveat

Sheldon and Lyubomirsky (2006) recommend doing the Best Possible Self exercise over 4 weeks rather than as a once-off writing activity. It is important to view this exercise as part of your "sustainable happiness" activities (Lyubomirsky et al., 2005; Sheldon & Lyubomirsky, 2004) and not a once-off action. We are more likely to do exercises like this if we expect to enjoy them and if the activity resonates with us. So the value of this exercise will depend on how much it fits with what you like to do usually.

References

Cameron, L. D., & Nicholls, G. (1998). Expression of stressful experiences through writing: Effects of a self regulation manipulation for pessimists and optimists. *Health Psychology, 17,* 84–92.

Carrillo, A., Etchemendy, E., & Baños, R. M. (2021). My best self in the past, present or future: Results of two randomized controlled trials. *Journal of Happiness Studies, 22*(2), 955–980. https://doi-org.elib.tcd.ie/10.1007/s10902-020-00259-z

Emmons, R. A. (1986). Personal strivings: An approach to personality and subjective wellbeing. *Journal of Personality and Social Psychology, 51,* 1058–1068.

Gibson, B., Umeh, K., Davies, I., & Newson, L. (2021). The best possible self-intervention as a viable public health tool for the prevention of type 2 diabetes: A reflexive thematic analysis of public experience and engagement. *Health Expectations: An International Journal of Public Participation in Health Care and Health Policy, 24*(5), 1713–1724. https://doi.org/10.1111/hex.13311

King, L. A. (2001). The health benefits of writing about life goals. *Personality and Social Psychology Bulletin, 27*(7), 798–807.

King, L. A., & Miner, K. N. (2000). Writing about the perceived benefits of traumatic events: Implications for physical health. *Personality and Social Psychology Bulletin.* https://doi.org/10.1177/0146167200264008.

Lyubomirsky, S., Sheldon, K. M., & Schkade, D. (2005). Pursuing happiness: The architecture of sustainable change. *Review of General Psychology, 9,* 111–131.

Markus, H., & Nurius, P. (1986). Possible selves. *American psychologist, 41*(9), 954.

Omodei, M. M., & Wearing, A. J. (1990). Need satisfaction and involvement in personal projects: Toward an integrative model of subjective wellbeing. *Journal of Personality and Social Psychology, 59,* 762–769.

Rivkin, I. D., & Taylor, S. E. (1999). The effects of mental simulation on coping with controllable stressful events. *Personality and Social Psychology Bulletin, 25*, 1451–1462.

Round, J., & Burke, J. (2018). A dream of a retirement: The longitudinal experiences and perceived retirement wellbeing of recent retirees following a tailored intervention linking best possible self-expressive writing with goal-setting. *International Coaching Psychology Review, 13*(2), 27–45.

Sheldon, K. M., & Lyubomirsky, S. (2004). Achieving sustainable new happiness: Prospects, practices, and prescriptions. In A. Linley & S. Joseph (Eds.), *Positive psychology in practice* (pp. 127–145). John Wiley & Sons.

Sheldon, K. M., & Lyubomirsky, S. (2006). How to increase and sustain positive emotion: The effects of expressing gratitude and visualizing best possible selves. *The Journal of Positive Psychology, 1*(2), 73–82. doi:10.1080/17439760500510676

Hope

When everything else fails, hope prevails. Without hope, we cannot get up, dust ourselves off, and keep going. Hope is an essential ingredient for coping. The difference between optimism and hope is significant. Optimism gives us the expectation that everything will work out well. Hope, however, gives us the will and the way to keep going in a specific direction. It is a mixture of agency thinking and clear pathway thinking that helps us get there (Snyder, 1994). Agency thinking is about maintaining the energy to pursue our dreams and goals and keep the motivation going. It is about saying to ourselves that we can do it, we have all it takes to do it, and firmly believing that we can keep going, even when we face obstacles. Pathway thinking relates to developing a clear route towards accomplishing our goals. For example, it is not enough to say that you want to become a famous singer. Instead, to create a pathway, we need to develop a route for getting there: attending voice classes, practising daily, signing up to a choir, and similar activities. When we have the goal and the pathway towards it developed and then have the agency thinking clarified, we will experience hope. Thus, hope is far from wishful thinking. It is, in fact, the opposite. It is a plan and a belief that we have what it takes to sustain the energy to keep going and ultimately reach it.

Research-based tools

Tool 108: Hope profiling (adapted from Lopez et al., 2004)

Write five stories about your past or current goal pursuits. As you write your stories, please include information about how you developed your goals or paths you followed in working toward your goal and where your motivation to work on your goals came from. Feel free to write about goal pursuits in your various life domains.

Create three columns on your paper. On the top of the first column, write "Goals"; on the top of the second column, write "Pathways"; on the top of the third column, write "Obstacles". Under Goals, write down a goal for using one of your strengths (see the Strengths tools). In the Pathways column, write down at least three ways in which you can accomplish your goal or make using your strengths easier. In the Obstacles column, write down at least one obstacle for each pathway you mentioned.

PART 2

Reflect on how you will keep your motivation for accomplishing your goal. Who can help you do it? What other resources can you activate to make it happen?

Variations of practice

There are over 20 definitions and many different models of hope (e.g. Averill et al., 1990; Gottschalk, 1985). Nonetheless, the most frequently used model comprises agency and pathway thinking (Snyder, 1994). Therefore, many interventions follow its structure. This can be done as a facilitation session (as short as a 90-minute engagement) with a group of people or as a coaching session with a client. It follows a structure of finding a realistic goal, exploring a range of ways to reach it, including potential obstacles, and considering the type of positive talk we can engage in to help us maximise our potential, commitment, and motivation (Chan et al., 2019).

Some researchers suggest that watching hopeful films can indeed inspire us to feel hopeful about the future (Niemiec & Wedding, 2014), which may, in turn, inspire us to "think" hopeful thoughts about our lives. Similarly, in a controlled experiment with 60 participants exposed to "positive music", it seems that music increased their hopeful state compared with those who did not listen to music (Ziv et al., 2011). This experiment was conducted as part of a dissertation; however, it was not published in a peer-reviewed journal. Nonetheless, if you wish to experiment with your psyche, you may choose to listen to positive tunes and decide whether it enhances your wellbeing.

Check out other tools in this book

The Best Possible Self activity is most frequently used for enhancing optimism and hope (Loveday et al., 2018). Also, please review the section about Goal Setting.

Mental and physical health benefits

Hope interventions have been tested with people of all ages, professions, and various depictions of health. Hope-enhanced participants' positive emotions lead to upward spirals of positivity that result in a range of positive outcomes, such as wellbeing. Furthermore, those who reported higher levels of hope before 9/11 showed a significant increase of hope afterwards (Fredrickson et al., 2003), indicating the intricate nature of hope, the experiences of which multiply in the face of adversity.

Hope is instrumental in palliative care to help terminally ill patients come to terms with their fate (Gum & Snyder, 2002). Despite its apparent conflict, it respects individuals' autonomy and contributes to their welfare (Garrard & Wrigley, 2009). It is also fundamental for individuals diagnosed with a potentially fatal illness, such as cancer; it results in experiencing less distress and demonstrating more adaptive coping (Taylor, 2000). On a practical level, it prompts solution search and pursuit to improve their chances of survival. A review of the literature relating to the experiences of hope among adolescent patients with chronic illness found that it promotes such outcomes as health and effective coping and improves the quality of life, self-esteem, and resilience (Griggs & Walker, 2016). Among cancer patients, even a short intervention helped them enhance their hope and reduce symptoms of depression (Chan et al., 2019). From the physiological perspective, dispositional hope is associated with a higher pain threshold (Snyder et al., 2005). Furthermore, several studies were carried out with individuals with spinal cord injury showing that sustaining hope amid their life changes increased their motivation to keep going and life satisfaction (Yui et al., 2013). Thus, having hope is helpful in healthcare settings.

Caveats

Don't expect miracles after doing a short intervention for enhancing hope. Most of the interventions are long term, thus allowing participants to go through a process of enhancing hope over time. After all, hope is an outcome of thinking, not only a fleeting emotion.

Please note that hoping for something implausible to happen, e.g. giving birth to a child when a woman is over 55 (blocked goal), does not relate to the experience of hope as we described it.

References

Averill, J. R., Catlin, G., & Chon, K. K. (1990). *Rules of hope*. Springer-Verlag Publishing. https://doi.org/10.1007/978-1-4613-9674-1

Chan, K., Wong, F. K. Y., & Lee, P. H. (2019). A brief hope intervention to increase hope level and improve well-being in rehabilitating cancer patients: A feasibility test. *SAGE Open Nursing*. https://doi.org/10.1177/2377960819844381

Fredrickson, B. L., Tugade, M. M., Waugh, C. E., & Larkin, G. R. (2003). What good are positive emotions in crises? A prospective study of resilience and emotions following the terrorist attacks on the United States on September 11th, 2001. *Journal of Personality and Social Psychology, 84*(2), 365–376. https://doi.org/10.1037//0022-3514.84.2.365

Garrard, E., & Wrigley, A. (2009). Hope and terminal illness: False hope versus absolute hope. *Clinical Ethics, 4*(1), 38–43. https://doi-org.elib.tcd.ie/10.1258/ce.2008.008050

Gottschalk, L. A. (1985). Hope and other deterrents to illness. *American Journal of Psychotherapy, 39*(4), 515–524.

Griggs, S., & Walker, R. K. (2016). The role of hope for adolescents with a chronic illness: An integrative review. *Journal of Pediatric Nursing, 31*(4), 404–421. https://doi.org/10.1016/j.pedn.2016.02.011

Gum, A., & Snyder, C. R. (2002). Coping with terminal illness: The role of hopeful thinking. *Journal of Palliative Medicine, 5*(6), 883–894. https://doi-org.elib.tcd.ie/10.1089/10966210260499078

Lopez, S. J., Snyder, C. R., Magyar-Moe, J. L., Edwards, L. M., Pedrotti, J. T., Janowski, K., Turner, J. L., & Pressgrove, C. (2004). Strategies for accentuating hope. In P. A. Linley & S. Joseph (Eds.), *Positive psychology in practice* (pp. 388–404). John Wiley & Sons, Inc.

Loveday, P. M., Lovell, G. P., & Jones, C. M. (2018). The best possible selves intervention: A review of the literature to evaluate efficacy and guide future research. *Journal of Happiness Studies: An Interdisciplinary Forum on Subjective Well-Being, 19*(2), 607–628. https://doi-org.elib.tcd.ie/10.1007/s10902-016-9824-z

Niemiec, R., & Wedding, D. (2014). *Positive psychology at the movies 2: Using films to build character strengths and wellbeing* (2nd ed.). Hogreffe.

Snyder, C. R. (1994). *The psychology of hope: You can get there from here*. Free Press.

Snyder, C. R., Berg, C., Woodward, J. T., Gum, A., Rand, K. L., Wrobleski, K. K., Brown, J., & Hackman, A. (2005). Hope against the cold: Individual differences in trait hope and acute pain tolerance on the cold pressor task. *Journal of Personality, 73*(2), 287–312. https://doi-org.elib.tcd.ie/10.1111/j.1467-6494.2005.00318.x

Taylor, J. D. (2000). Confronting breast cancer: Hopes for health. In C. R. Snyder (Ed.), *Handbook of hope: Theory, measures, and applications* (pp. 355–371). Academic Press. https://doi-org.elib.tcd.ie/10.1016/B978-012654050-5/50021-X

Yui Chung Chan, J., Fong Chan, Ditchman, N., Phillips, B., & Chih-Chin Chou. (2013). Evaluating Snyder's hope theory as a motivational model of participation and life satisfaction for individuals with spinal cord injury: A path analysis. *Rehabilitation Research, Policy & Education*, 27(3), 171–185. https://doi-org.elib.tcd.ie/10.1891/2168-6653.27.3.171

Ziv, N., Ben Haim, A., & Itamar, O. (2011). The effect of positive music and dispositional hope on state hope and affect. *Psychology of Music*, 39(1), 3–17.

Your reflection space

Which prospecting tools would you like to try? Why?
Which activities did you find most useful? How did you tweak them?

9 Emerging tools and concepts

Whilst in this book, we focused on presenting tools that provide research on their impact on mental, physical, and physiological health, as well as research carried out with clinical and non-clinical populations, there are several tools and concepts which, despite lacking one or more criteria for inclusion for this book, can prove very helpful for enhancing wellbeing. These are either concepts without tested tools or interventions with insufficient research. We are flagging them as a way of encouraging you to read more about them or try them out anyway. Who knows; they could work for you.

Storytelling

Whether it's the warmth and depth of a good novel, the thrills of an action movie, the plot twists of a binge-able TV show, or a colleague relaying some juicy gossip, we all love a good story. We seem to be hardwired to listen to or tell stories as a species. In Ireland, the Seanchaí (pronounced shan-a-key) are storytellers who, in the past, travelled the countryside with their stories for bread and board. The Seanchaí kept oral traditions alive in Ireland, and there are cultural equivalents worldwide. These storytellers were much respected and valued in the community. Although we understand anecdotally that telling or receiving a story can make us feel good, up until recently, there has been little scientific evidence to confirm what we already instinctively feel. In 2021, Brockington and co-workers tested the power of storytelling on the psychological and physiological wellbeing of 81 children attending the intensive care unit of a Brazilian hospital. This was a randomised controlled study with an active control group, where children were offered a riddle instead of a story for up to 30 minutes. The other group received a 30-minute story from experienced storytellers. The results showed that the stress hormone cortisol was reduced in the saliva of these children.

DOI: 10.4324/9781003279594-11

In contrast, the hormone associated with human connection and love, oxytocin, was significantly increased after listening to each story (compared with children from the active control group). Furthermore, storytelling increased positive emotions and reduced pain perception among these children (Brockington et al., 2021). This is just one study looking at sick children. However, it might be the first of many proving what we instinctively feel – storytelling is powerful and can make us feel well.

Try this

Immerse yourself in listening to stories and find opportunities to share stories with others.

Self-care

We have always instinctively known that how we look is associated with wellbeing. For example, museums worldwide display jewellery of people living in prehistoric times for whom everything they owned mattered; tribes worldwide use jewellery to differentiate themselves from other tribes, become more attractive to potential partners, or assert power. What we wear and how we wear it is a form of self-expression and a medium for constructing our social identity; it communicates essential information about us; for example, our gender, age, conformity, rebelliousness. It also has a significant impact on our emotions, thoughts, and behaviours, which may originate from self or the feedback we receive from others (e.g. people smiling, looking at us with approval, or commenting on how we look). Sometimes we can choose our image, e.g. choose the clothes, shoes, or perfume we wear; other times, our image may be or feel out of our control, e.g. scarring or hair loss due to cancer or alopecia. In summary, self-care is not just about aesthetics and vanity but an intricate psychological process that can significantly impact our emotions, thoughts and identity.

Adam and Galinsky (2012) coined the term "enclothed cognition", which describes clothes' impact on our psychological processes. Their experiment found that when scientists wore a lab coat when performing their duties, they paid more attention to their work. An experiment with nurses wearing or not wearing a nursing tunic demonstrated similar results impacting their empathetic and altruistic behaviour (López-Pérez et al., 2016). In the same way, as we may embody our emotions, we can enclothe our thinking. However, enclothed cognition is a new concept, and despite many studies showing similar results, it is also met with some criticism (e.g. Burns et al., 2019). We need more research to understand the causal effects further.

Most of the studies about "wearing wellbeing" is non-experimental. There is a clear indication in the literature that what we wear is associated with wellbeing; however, we don't know whether we choose clothes and shoes and jewellery based on how we feel or aspire to feel or whether they indeed make us feel better. More research is required to include this as a tool in this book.

While we wait for research to catch up with common sense, do whatever makes you happy. Self-care refers to any form of caring for the body. This may be taking the time to do your hair, go to a barber, or do up someone else's hair. For example, in African culture, hair styling is seen as psychotherapy, with mothers and daughters bonding with each other while styling their hair (Mbilishaka et al., 2021). For people with depression, just putting on clothes can be seen as a great accomplishment that can help them feel better. Wearing makeup is associated with enhanced levels of self-reported wellbeing, self-esteem, and self-confidence (Fares et al., 2019; Kosmala et al., 2019). A single makeup session and an upper-body photoshoot reduced the symptoms of depression and enhanced the quality of life and self-esteem of women with early breast cancer, and the change continued at moderate levels 8 weeks post-intervention (Richard et al., 2019).

Try this

Fun shoes: Next time you buy shoes, buy shoes that make you smile, shoes that turn other people's heads around. One of our colleagues prided herself upon her unique shoe collection. She loved wearing unusual, patterned shoes. Shoes that looked different felt different and matched her mood. She talked about the joy of deciding what shoes to wear and the happiness she experienced looking down at them throughout the day. However, the most significant positive boost for her was the social connection she received as strangers smiled at her or started a conversation about her unusual shoes.

Dress up: What you wear is associated with your mood. During COVID-19, many of us worked from home, and it was easy to stay in a dressing gown for the day or wear the PJ bottoms while attending an important meeting. However, dressing up can sometimes make us feel better. So why not try getting dressed up nicely for yourself? Even if you are staying at home for the day, put on nice clothes and watching your mood pick up.

Social media

Many years ago, one of my clients felt lonely. His life revolved around his family and work. Soon, the monotony of his daily existence resulted in a low mood, frustration, and loneliness. One of the suggestions we discussed was engaging with social media to help him reconnect with others. He, therefore, began a picture-a-day project whereby instead of having a sandwich at his desk, he went outside during his lunch hour, took a picture of nature or anything else that caught his attention, and posted it online with a brief comment. Soon, his pictures became a daily activity that brought him lots of enjoyment, and as he was receiving many "likes" and comments, he began to feel more connected to others. This also resulted in a few of his old friends writing private messages and arranging a catch-up. Within a month from the beginning of his project, he gleamed, reflecting on how much his life had changed for the better. When used responsibly, engaging with social media can be helpful. However, overusing social media can also have a negative effect.

Social media is defined as informal online activities that share information using pictures, audio, words, and videos (Welch et al., 2016). They include blogs and microblogs, such as Twitter, content communities, such as YouTube, discussion groups, interactive apps, virtual gaming worlds, and virtual social networks, such as Facebook.

Spending too much time on social media is not suitable for our wellbeing. Yet abstinence from it is associated with higher levels of loneliness, more experiences of negative emotions, and a decline in life satisfaction (Vally & D'Souza, 2019). Thus, a happy medium of engaging with online resources is recommended. Furthermore, social media can help people connect. This is pertinent, especially when we go through difficult times. For example, patients diagnosed with cancer or autism found connecting with like groups particularly useful, which resulted in their being more informed about their condition and resources available to them as well as making them feel less lonely and more supported (Falisi et al., 2017; Ward et al., 2018).

Furthermore, social media can be particularly beneficial for those who lack social skills to develop social capital, as they can engage with others, share their opinion, and receive support in the absence of a conventional face-to-face relationship (Ziv & Kiasi, 2015). The impact of social media engagement on wellbeing is nuanced. While many studies identify increases in various aspects of wellbeing, such as relationships with others, other studies warn about its negative impact, especially when overused (Gudka et al., 2021). The increase in wellbeing among those who use social media is attributed to two factors. Social media may result in harmful comparison, whereby comparing self with other's fortune is amplified online and results in wellbeing decline (Reer et al., 2019). Given that persistent users experienced higher comparison levels, it is recommended to reduce engagement with social media when we begin to experience negative emotions. Also, a systematic review of research relating to social media use and eating disorder found that the frequency of use and image sharing impacts symptoms of eating disorders (Friero et al., 2021); therefore, care needs to be taken to moderate usages in these circumstances and engage with text-based instead of image-based social media.

Try this

Social media break: When you feel that social media begins to have a negative impact on you, or you started to feel unwell recently and consider yourself a frequent social media user, stop using it for a week (Brown & Kuss, 2020) or abstain from using your phone shortly before going to bed (Hughes & Burke, 2018) and assess if it positively impacts your wellbeing. Then, modulate your behaviour accordingly to ensure that social media doesn't get in the way of your wellbeing.

Support group: Find an online group that helps you feel connected to people whose experience is similar to yours (Williams, 2014). For example, if you have been recently diagnosed with an illness or are interested in hiking, find a group that will help you get you all the information you need about it.

Harmonious passion

Sometimes passion is overrated. When in school, children are encouraged to search for passion and told they will never be bored again; passionate activities will come easily and make them successful. Employees are promised the same at work, with the addition that work will never feel like work again when they find passion. Yet research indicates that when people are passionate about something, be it what they do for a living or a hobby, they are less likely to put effort into delving deeper into the activity. As a result, such passion may prevent them from developing their expertise and ultimately reaching success (O'Keefe et al., 2018). This happens due to an implicit belief that passion means that what they do should keep them interested and, hence, does not require extra effort. This is also one of the reasons some people keep changing their passion, and as soon as they lose interest, they think that they were mistaken about calling it passion. Or they may say that their passion is short-lived.

Additionally, researchers recognise that while some passions (harmonious) enhance our physical health and psychological wellbeing, other types of passions (obsessive) make us miserable (Vallerand et al., 2003). When passion is obsessive, individuals become fixated on developing their passion, to the extent that thinking about it makes them experience negative emotions. On the other hand, when their passion is harmonious, they can experience full engagement in this and other activities, whilst working on developing their passion results mostly in experiencing positive emotions.

For example, imagine that your recent passion is preparing for a marathon. You have never done this before, and you are committed to accomplishing it. If your passion is obsessive, likely, you will significantly reduce other enjoyable activities in your life, such as meeting up with friends or having that favourite meal. Apart from those that help you prepare for a marathon, you may experience more guilt when engaging in other activities. Furthermore, your pride will make you persevere through pain to an extent that you may have damaged your ligaments, yet instead of taking the time out to recuperate, you will keep going. You will keep on focusing on what other people will think of you if you don't do it, and this will keep your motivation going.

On the other hand, you may be harmoniously passionate about running a marathon, meaning that while you will be training for it more, you will also maintain balance and keep another hobby in your life. You will not feel guilty about taking a respite, especially when you notice that something is not okay with your body. If you experience any injury, you will go to the doctor and, if needed, forgo the marathon. Most importantly, you will enjoy the process, and seeing it as a personal accomplishment will be your biggest motivator.

While we have a lot of research suggesting a strong relationship between harmonious passion and wellbeing, there are no tested interventions to help us move into the healthier passion mindset.

Try this

Whenever you find yourself obsessing about something you love, to the extent that it makes you feel bad about yourself, stop and reflect on what changes you can make to make your passion more harmonious.

Self-reassurance

Reassuring yourself is an activity that involves talking to yourself from a perspective of care and compassion. It is the opposite of self-criticism.

In self-reassurance, the aim is not to counter or critique your thinking but rather to be understanding and compassionate towards your negative thoughts (Petrocchi et al., 2018). The ability to self-reassure is related to increased resilience and psychological wellbeing (Trompetter et al., 2017). It is negatively correlated with depression in clinical and non-clinical research groups (Petrocchi et al., 2018). Gilbert et al. (2008) argue that the ability to self-reassure is implicated in the positive emotional experience of feeling safe and content. Their study showed that the safe and content positive emotion "had the highest negative correlations with depression, anxiety and stress, self-criticism and insecure attachment" (p. 182). In functional MRI studies, self-reassurance has been shown to stimulate brain regions to express compassion and empathy towards others (Lutz et al., 2008). In terms of psychological health, there is some indirect evidence (Rockliff et al., 2008) that self-reassurance and the self-compassion it evokes positively affect the parasympathetic nervous system, triggering the rest-and-digest response, helping people feel safe and contented (Kirby et al., 2017).

Try this

When things don't go your way in life, it is essential to practice self-reassurance; you can do it by having a compassionate attitude toward yourself, filled with encouragement and reminding yourself of all your assets, strengths, qualities, and skills you can use in the face of adversity (Petrocchi et al., 2018). Also, loving-kindness meditation is a way to develop self-reassurance, a form of self-compassion. If you struggle to be good at self-reassurance, the loving-kindness meditation can help you do it.

Finally, reducing self-criticism is part of developing the skill of self-reassurance. Research has shown that writing about your best possible self reduces our self-critical voice (Troop et al., 2013) and facilitates self-assurance. If you struggle to be good at self-reassurance and do not like meditation, the expressive writing Best Possible Self is a good starting point.

Self-reassurance is an approach used in compassion-focused therapy. It is different from the challenging negative thoughts activity used in cognitive behavioural therapy. Both methods have their benefits, so it's important not to dismiss one over the other. Still, it is worth considering that self-reassurance is particularly beneficial for highly self-critical people (Petrocchi et al., 2018).

References

Adam, H., & Galinsky, A. D. (2012). Enclothed cognition. *Journal of Experimental Social Psychology*, *48*(4), 918–925. https://doi.org/10.1016/j.jesp.2012.02.008

Brockington, G., Gomes Moreira, A. P., Buso, M. S., Gomes da Silva, S., Altszyler, E., Fischer, R., & Moll, J. (2021). Storytelling increases oxytocin and positive emotions and decreases cortisol and pain in hospitalized children. *Proceedings of the National Academy of Sciences*, *118*(22), e2018409118. doi:10.1073/pnas.2018409118

Burns, D. M., Fox, E. L., Greenstein, M., Olbright, G., & Montgomery, D. (2019). An old task in new clothes: A preregistered direct replication attempt of enclothed cognition effects on Stroop performance. *Journal of Experimental Social Psychology*, *83*, 150–156. https://doi-org.elib.tcd.ie/10.1016/j.jesp.2018.10.001

Falisi, A., Wiseman, K., Gaysynsky, A., Scheideler, J., Ramin, D., Chou, W., Falisi, A. L., Wiseman, K. P., Scheideler, J. K., Ramin, D. A., & Chou, W.-Y. S. (2017). Social media for breast cancer survivors: A literature review. *Journal of Cancer Survivorship*, *11*(6), 808–821. https://doi-org.elib.tcd.ie/10.1007/s11764-017-0620-5

Fares, K., Hallit, S., Haddad, C., Akel, M., Khachan, T., & Obeid, S. (2019). Relationship between cosmetics use, self-esteem, and self-perceived attractiveness among Lebanese women. *Journal of Cosmetic Science*, *70*(1), 47–56.

Friero, P., González-Rodríguez, R., Verde-Diego, C., & Vázquez-Pérez, R. (2021). Social media and eating disorder psychopathology: A systematic review. *Cyberpsychology*, *15*(3), 1–21. https://doi-org.elib.tcd.ie/10.5817/CP2021-3-6

Gilbert, P., McEwan, K., Mitra, R., Franks, L., Richter, A., & Rockliff, H. (2008). Feeling safe and content: A specific affect regulation system? Relationship to depression, anxiety, stress, and self-criticism. *The Journal of Positive Psychology*, *3*(3), 182–191. doi:10.1080/17439760801999461

Gudka, M., Gardiner, K. L. K., & Lomas, T. (2021). Towards a framework for flourishing through social media: A systematic review of 118 research studies. *The Journal of Positive Psychology*. https://doi-org.elib.tcd.ie/10.1080/17439760.2021.1991447

Hughes, N., & Burke, J. (2018). Sleeping with the frenemy: How restricting 'bedroom use' of smartphones impacts happiness and wellbeing. *Computers in Human Behavior*, *85*, 236–244. https://doi-org.elib.tcd.ie/10.1016/j.chb.2018.03.047

Kirby, J., & Gilbert, P. (2017). The emergence of the compassion focused therapies. In P. Gilbert (Ed.), *Compassion: Concepts, research and applications* (pp. 258–285). Routledge.

Kosmala, A., Wilk, I., & Kassolik, K. (2019). Influence of makeup on the wellbeing and self-esteem of women. *Pielęgniarstwo i Zdrowie Publiczne Nursing and Public Health*, *9*(3), 215–220. doi:10.17219/pzp/105811

López-Pérez, B., Ambrona, T., Wilson, E. L., & Khalil, M. (2016). The effect of enclothed cognition on empathic responses and helping behavior. *Social Psychology*, *47*(4), 223–231. https://doi-org.elib.tcd.ie/10.1027/1864-9335/a000273

Lutz, A., Brefczynski-Lewis, J., Johnstone, T., & Davidson, R. J. (2008). Regulation of the theme neural circuitry of emotion by compassion meditation: Effects of the meditative expertise. *Public Library of Science One*, *3*, 1–5. https://doi-org.proxy.library.rcsi.ie/10.1371/journal.pone.0001897

Mbilishaka, A. M., Mbande, A., Gulley, C., & Mbande, T. (2021). Faded fresh tapers and line-ups: Centering barbershop hair stories in understanding gendered racial socialization for black men. *Psychology of Men & Masculinities*, *22*(1), 166–176. https://doi.org/10.1037/men0000317

O'Keefe, P. A., Dweck, C. S., & Walton, G. M. (2018). Implicit theories of interest: Finding your passion or developing it? *Psychological Science, 29*(10), 1653–1664. https://doi-org.elib.tcd.ie/10.1177/0956797618780643

Petrocchi, N., Dentale, F., & Gilbert, P. (2018). Self-reassurance, not self-esteem, serves as a buffer between self-criticism and depressive symptoms. *Psychology and Psychotherapy: Theory, Research and Practice, 92*(3), 394–406. https://doi-org.proxy.library.rcsi.ie/10.1111/papt.12186

Reer, F., Tang, W. Y., & Quandt, T. (2019). Psychosocial wellbeing and social media engagement: The mediating roles of social comparison orientation and fear of missing out. *New Media & Society, 21*(7), 1486–1505. https://doi.org/10.1177/1461444818823719

Richard, A., Harbeck, N., Wuerstlein, R., & Wilhelm, F. H. (2019). Recover your smile: Effects of a beauty care intervention on depressive symptoms, quality of life, and self-esteem in patients with early breast cancer. *Psycho-Oncology, 28*(2), 401–407. https://doi-org.elib.tcd.ie/10.1002/pon.4957

Rockliff, H., Gilbert, P., McEwan, K., Lightman, S., & Glover, D. (2008). A pilot exploration of heart rate variability and salivary cortisol responses to compassion-focused imagery. *Clinical Neuropsychiatry: Journal of Treatment Evaluation, 5*(3), 132–139. https://derby.openrepository.com/bitstream/handle/10545/622861/McEwan_2008_A_pilot_exploration_of_heart_rate_variability_and_salivary_cortisol_responses_to_compassion_focused_imagery_published.pdf?sequence=6&isAllowed=y

Trompetter, H. R., Kleine, E., & de Bohlmeijer, E. T. (2017). Why does positive mental health buffer against psychopathology? An exploratory study on self-compassion as a resilience mechanism and adaptive emotion regulation strategy. *Cognitive Therapy and Research, 41*, 459–468. https://doi-org.proxy.library.rcsi.ie/10.1007/s10608-016-9774-0

Troop, N. A., Chilcot, J., Hutchings, L., & Varnaite, G. (2013). Expressive writing, self-criticism, and self-reassurance. *Psychology and Psychotherapy: Theory, Research and Practice, 86*, 374–386. https://doi-org.proxy.library.rcsi.ie/10.1111/j.2044-8341.2012.02065.x

Vallerand, R. J., Blanchard, C., Mageau, G. A., Koestner, R., Ratelle, C., Leonard, M., Gagne, M., & Marsolais, J. (2003). Les passions de l'ame: on obsessive and harmonious passion. *Journal of Personality and Social Psychology, 85*(4), 756–767. https://doi-org.elib.tcd.ie/10.1037/0022-3514.85.4.756

Vally, Z., & D'Souza, C. G. (2019). Abstinence from social media use, subjective well-being, stress, and loneliness. *Perspectives in Psychiatric Care, 55*(4), 752–759. https://doi-org.elib.tcd.ie/10.1111/ppc.12431

Ward, D. M., Dill-Shackleford, K. E., & Mazurek, M. O. (2018). Social media use and happiness in adults with autism spectrum disorder. *Cyberpsychology, Behavior, and Social Networking, 21*(3), 205–209. https://doi-org.elib.tcd.ie/10.1089/cyber.2017.0331

Welch, V., Petkovic, J., Pardo, J., Rader, T., & Tugwell, P. (2016). Interactive social media interventions to promote health equity: An overview of reviews. *Health Promotion and Chronic Disease Prevention in Canada: Research, Policy and Practice, 36*(4), 63–75. https://doi.org/10.24095/hpcdp.36.4.01

Williams, B. (2014). Group therapy: A natural opportunity for support. *Practice Nursing*, *25*(4), 190–194.

Ziv, I., & Kiasi, M. (2016). Facebook's contribution to wellbeing among adolescent and young adults as a function of mental resilience. *The Journal of Psychology: Interdisciplinary and Applied*, *150*(4), 527–541. https://doi-org.elib.tcd.ie/10.1080/002 23980.2015.1110556

Part III
Making a lasting change

10 Going with the waves of change

Change is not easy. Even if you are fully motivated to enhance your health and wellbeing, you buy this book, select your health and wellbeing activities, and approach them with a gung-ho attitude, you may still find it challenging to achieve your goals. There are many reasons for this, and in this section, we will discuss some of the main obstacles that may get in the way of your success. Familiarising yourself with potential obstacles will help you prepare for them and hopefully overcome them more effectively.

When creating the list of obstacles and potential solutions to them, we have drawn on over half a century of the theories developed by psychologists to help you change your behaviour, engage more effectively with wellbeing and health tools, and maintain your behaviour. Table 10.1 provides a list of the theories this chapter is based on. Feel free to review it further if you are interested in learning more. In the meantime, let's get to work and tackle those obstacles that get in the way of you changing and maintaining your new health and wellbeing practice.

"I don't know how to improve my health and wellbeing" or *"I know what I need to do, I just don't know where to start"*.

Reading this book will give you the knowledge on how to do it, and this chapter will hopefully provide you with the steps you can take to apply your knowledge. If this doesn't work, you can work with a health coach or a therapist who would guide you through the process of skills improvement. Alternatively, you can reflect on how you have built your skills in the past. What has worked for you? Who did you do it with? What resources have you used? Then, come up with a plan to apply the same technique to improve your health and wellbeing skills.

"I am not sure if I am ready to improve my health and wellbeing now. Maybe next year".

DOI: 10.4324/9781003279594-13

Table 10.1 Behavioural change theories applied in this book to help you change health and wellbeing behaviour and maintain it.

Theory	Brief description
Operant Learning Theory (Skinner, 1953)	All behaviour has consequences. Positive consequences will encourage you to keep going. Punishment will lead only to a temporary change, and soon, you will revert to unwanted behaviour. This theory favours positive reinforcement. E.g. *Treat yourself after completing a difficult tool.*
Social Learning Theory (Bandura, 1971)	We live in a social world, and as such, we can learn from others. Model other people's behaviour, break it down into sequence and practice. E.g. *do you know someone who walks every day for 1 hour? How do they do it? How do they find the time, and what do they do when it's raining? Ask them, observe them, figure out how they overcome obstacles, and try it out yourself.*
Social Cognitive Theory (Bandura, 1997)	Self-efficacy is our confidence to make changes or perform certain tasks. Our confidence increases via four sources: (1) mastery experiences, (2) modelling, (3) social/verbal persuasion, and (4) physiological experiences. E.g. *I'm not sure if I can enhance my wellbeing. To improve my self-efficacy, I keep practising tools (mastery), I watch how my friend engages with tools and can already see a positive change in her (modelling). My friend cheers me on (verbal persuasion), and I had butterflies in my stomach when doing some of the tools. I thought I was anxious, but now I know I was just excited.*
Theory of Planned Behaviour (Ajzen, 1991)	Our intentions are determined by a mixture of our (1) attitude towards the behaviour, (2) social norms, and (3) how much we can control the behaviour. E.g. *your success in weight loss will depend on your attitude towards it (losing weight will make me healthier), social norms (as a family, we eat a lot of fast food), perceived control (I will not be able to stop myself when my family gets a take-away).*
Health Action Process Approach (Schwarzer, 1992)[1]	Forming a goal is not enough to change behaviour. After setting up a goal, we plan with task self-efficacy, coping self-efficacy, and recovery self-efficacy, and only then we act. E.g. *I would like to do expressive writing (goal). I plan the following. I am confident I have a good plan and can do this tool every day for the next 3 days (plan for task self-efficacy). Even when my life becomes hectic, I have a clear plan on how to keep going (plan for coping self-efficacy). However, if for whatever reason I stop doing this activity for a day or two, I have a plan on how to restart it (plan for recovery self-efficacy).*

Theory	Brief description
Transtheoretical model (Prochaska & DiClemente, 1983)	There are five distinct stages of behavioural change, (1) pre-contemplation (we do not consider a change), (2) contemplation (we consider pros and cons of change), (3) preparation (planning for a change), (4) action (taking steps to change), and (5) maintenance (sustaining changed behaviour). *E.g. I have read this book, and I'm considering doing something, but I am not yet sure if I am ready to engage with the tools; maybe in a few months (contemplation).*
Self-determination theory (Deci & Ryan, 1985)	Six types of motivation can influence your behaviour: (1) amotivation (we don't want to change), (2) external (to avoid punishment, others want us to do it), (3) introjected (we want to avoid negative emotions, e.g. feeling guilty), (4) identified (our behaviour will result in outcomes we value), (5) integrated (our behaviour is aligned with our values and identity, e.g. it feels right), and (6) intrinsic (we do it for its own sake, we enjoy it). The more you move towards intrinsic, the more likely you are to sustain your planned behaviour. *E.g. I should really use some of these activities to improve my wellbeing. It would be good not to feel so bad anymore (identified).*

If you are not ready to do it now, that's okay; you can leave it until next year. However, before you put this book aside, ask yourself why you chose to read this book in the first place. Ask yourself "why" many times (just like a child might), until you understand the deeper reasons for doing it. What has since changed? Can you make small changes for the time being that can serve you well? If so, what are they?

"I'm not sure I can change my health and wellbeing. I was born a pessimist".

Yes, we have a predisposition for wellbeing; however, it is not a life sentence, and you can still enhance it. We encourage you to re-read a section about genetic predisposition in Chapter 1. Hopefully, it will help you realise that you can do things to enhance your health and wellbeing, regardless of your age or personality.

"During the summer, I started a wellbeing-project, but as soon as I got back to work, I was too tired to continue. What if the same thing happens now?"

That was last year. Today can be different. Consider what you have learnt from your experience. What has worked for you? What has not that you would like to change?

"*Some tools just don't feel right.*"

If some tools don't feel right, don't use them. There are plenty of other tools that may be better suited to you. It is vital that the tools you have selected feel right. Otherwise, you will be less likely to engage with them. If there are tools that don't quite fit, try to tweak them to feel right. For example, if a tool asks you to take photographs and post them on social media, but you don't like using social media, then take photographs and create a little album in which you describe the meaning of each photograph. This may feel more "right" to you.

"*How do I select tools that suit my lifestyle?*"

Start by honestly assessing your schedule and then ruthlessly looking for a time to commit to yourself. You will choose tools that fit the time that you have available. Remember to try to push out that available time. Why is doing this tool vital to you? What is more important? What would you gain by doing this tool? And might you save time somewhere else if you take the time now to practice this tool? The other thing to consider is if you need any specific materials to do a tool, for example, writing material or a partner to forgive in the forgiveness exercise. And lastly, start with the easy tasks, the ones that fit with your life, and build up to ones that need may be more challenging.

"*My partner doesn't believe in psychology. If I started to count my blessings, he would laugh at me*".

What people who are essential in your life think of the changes you want to make is crucial and can significantly impact your success. If your partner, your friends, and other important people in your life do not agree with some of these activities, it can make your journey of change so much more difficult. You have two choices here. If the change is essential, brace yourself for some criticism and keep going. Becoming an authentic self is an arduous journey filled with many mixed emotions. Alternatively, you can select other tools that you may even try to do with others.

"*I don't have the time to read a book, let alone spend half an hour each day meditating or expressing myself in writing*".

That's a great point, and the beauty of this book is that you don't need half an hour each day; you don't even have to read the whole book! Some tools in here take as little as 5 to 10 minutes, and you can dip in and out of the tools and select individual tools without having to read the other ones.

"It's not me. I pride myself on my realism and criticism. I can't imagine myself completing a 'best possible self' activity. It's just too positive for me".

Yes, they are a bit too positive, and there's excellent value in realism. However, you can avoid these exercises altogether and still benefit from other exercises that best suit you. It might be interesting as a critical person to try these tasks for yourself and see how you respond to them. You can then thoroughly critique them, having tried them out!

"My family's favourite dinner is meat, potato, and veg. If I started to cook plant-based meals and give my children soy milk for their cereal, they wouldn't like it".

It's essential to keep the favourites going for your family. Small changes in meals might be a better way to go. Adding one new ingredient to the usual favourites or trying a soy-based dessert for fun could be an easy way in. Maybe your children will be moved by the meaning behind the changes if you ask them about their values and hopes for the environment and their health. Children often have more capacity for change than we give them credit for.

"I have great intentions, but when life gets busy, I stop looking after myself".

This is very common and normal. It is a great start that you notice this habit in yourself. This is the first step! Next time you are busy, you can try to be aware of this and make that the exact time to be mindful of looking after yourself. Looking after yourself is not optional; if you don't do it, you won't continue with your busy life. Start with tiny things: take 2 minutes for yourself to breathe or take a glass of water or be still. Notice you are busy and acknowledge the feeling. These are reasonable steps to stop the busy cycle and look after yourself.

"Will I be happier and healthier after I do these activities?"

Happiness is a subjective experience. We do not recommend that you do these activities to be happier. Pursuing happiness can make you self-focused and lonely. It is better to do these activities to maintain or enhance your wellbeing and health. However, there are no guarantees here. We hope that some of the activities in this book will help you do it. We have provided research-based tools that have helped many other people, so hopefully, they will help you too.

"My partner says I've been sad and irritable lately and that this book could help me. I'm not sure".

It is essential that you do this for yourself and not just because someone else wants you to change. It is also worth saying that being irritable and sad is okay and a normal part of the human experience. Do *you* think you need help?

"I value wellbeing and health, which is why I've read this book. What should I do next?"

Congratulations! Keep going; we never stop learning and growing. The first step is to solidify your identity as someone who values wellbeing and health. What steps support that identity? Who knows about this identity? Who in your circle would not be surprised to hear this about you? Can you find a community in which this identity can belong and thrive?

Reflection time

Having reviewed this section, what are your biggest challenges/obstacles for using the tools in this book to enhance your health and wellbeing?
What is your plan to overcome your challenges/obstacles?

Making positive change happen

Now that you have reflected on your obstacles, let us review ways to implement changes in your life after reading this book. These suggestions are not exhaustive, but they will at least get you started on your journey of improved health and wellbeing.

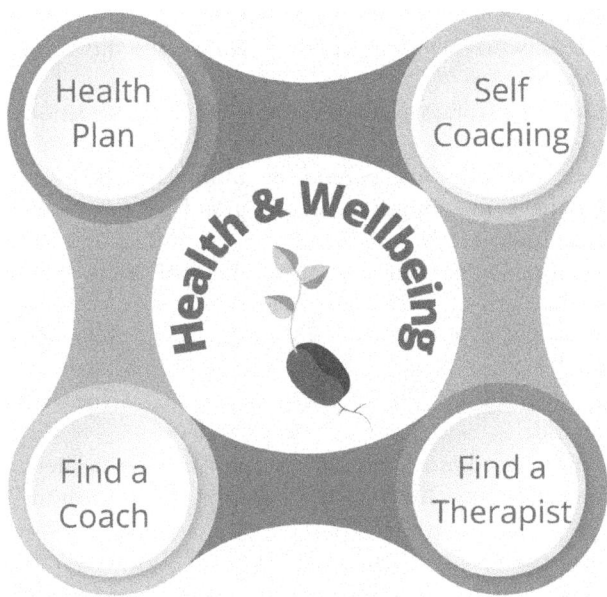

Figure 10.1 Four ways to enhance your health and wellbeing after reading this book.

Health plan

We all need help to sustain practices and develop habits and a new discipline. Luckily, researchers have investigated this for us. There are several best-practice guidelines in terms of helping you to maintain a sustainable habit. Researchers at University College London have shown that it takes, on average, 66 days to create a new habit (Lally et al., 2010). If you are one of the lucky ones, you will have a new habit within 22 days; for the rest, it might take up to 250 days. In short, it will take time, so hang in there.

After reading this book, you may be very clear about what you need to do. If so, you can start drawing up a health plan for yourself.

In terms of a plan, get your trusty pen and paper or phone, laptop, tablet (whatever suits you best) and put the following headings down:

- Identify barriers to your new habit and remove them (do not arrange a running schedule when you must drop the kids at school).

- Make your habit easy to follow (if running, keep your gear in the boot of your car).
- Try to keep your new practice to the same place and same time each day.
- Develop a new practice plan for the weekend, vacations, or trips away.
- Find out the meaning behind or motivation for your practice (e.g. I want to live longer to see my grandkids grow up) and write it out on paper.
- Tell everyone about your new plan – they will encourage you when needed.
- Piggyback the new habit on existing ones, e.g. floss after brushing your teeth.
- Follow SMART goals – specific, measurable, achievable, realistic, time bound.
- Have short-, medium-, and long-term goals – write them down.
- Have rewards for achieving each goal – short, medium, and long term.
- Get the support of a coach if needed.

This is an ongoing process. Hopefully, your written plan will become dog-eared and stained with use over time (hopefully). You will have to populate your headings. Become a detective. Be flexible and make alterations as you receive more information or your circumstances change. Incorporate the strategies listed in what follows of you can.

Use a coaching framework

Another way to embrace the content of this book is to use a coaching framework to plan for the change you would like to see. As we, the authors of this book, are all qualified in either coaching or therapy, we often apply some conversational frameworks to organise our thinking. We use a process with clients to figure out what next step we should take and how to go about it. A valuable tool for figuring out where to start is the Wheel of Change. It has been used extensively in the Quality of Life programme that helps individuals initiate health-related change (Frisch, 2006). We have adopted the wheel for this book and hope it will help you decide where to start. In Option 1, we introduce you to a Wheel of Health and Wellbeing that delves into all tools in this chapter. We offer you a process that allows you to decide what you want to focus on in Option 2.

Going with the waves of change 205

Option 1: the Wheel of Health and Wellbeing

This wheel is divided into eight parts representing each tool chapter of this book (Figure 10.2). Review each part and reflect on the following:

- How enjoyable and natural have you found the calming tools on a scale from 1 to 10?
  - Repeat this process for all other parts.
- Which one or two groups of tools would you find most helpful at this point? Please note they do not need to be tools you have scored the highest or the lowest in. Just the tools that "feel right" at this point.
- Briefly review the tools in this section and decide on or two tools you want to implement over the next week or a few weeks.

Please go to the next page, which will guide you through the goal-setting process.

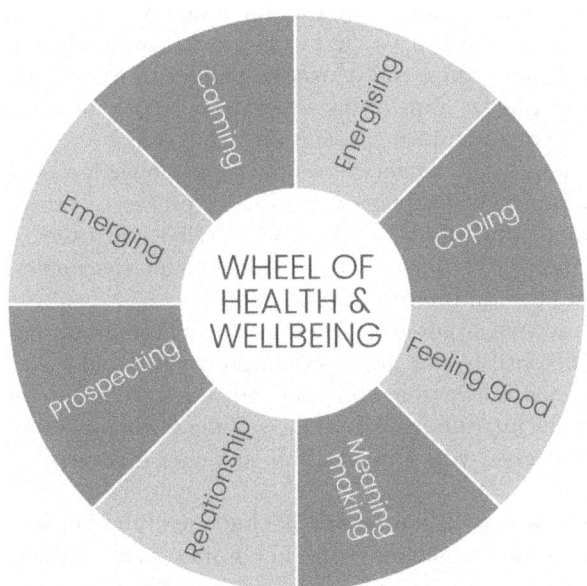

Figure 10.2 Wheel of Health and Wellbeing.

GROWTH framework

Effective coaching relies on structured conversational frameworks (van Nieuwerburgh, 2020). In other words, one reason coaching works is because coaches support their clients to bring about change by following a particular conversational process that increases the likelihood of success. Therefore, as you identify tools and approaches in this book that you would like to adopt, it may be helpful to follow such a process for yourself. One such model is the GROWTH framework (Campbell & van Nieuwerburgh, 2018), which is based on the original GROW model (Whitmore, 1992). GROWTH is an acronym that spells out the six stages: Goal, Reality/Resources, Options, Will, Tactics, and Habits. Each is explained in what follows.

- The first step is the Goal. What do you hope to achieve? Think through or write out what you would like to achieve. The more attractive this is, the more motivated you are likely to be. It is essential to give this attention, because the desired future goal will keep you going even if you face challenges later.
- The second step is to evaluate your current Reality and the resources you already have. Concerning your Goal, where are you now? Think through or write down your assessment of how close or far away you are from the Goal. If you're too close, the Goal might not be sufficiently motivating, and it may be helpful to reconsider the Goal. If you're too far away, think of some sub-goals or interim objectives on your way to the distant Goal and start by working towards them. This is also an excellent time to acknowledge what resources you have that will support you to make progress. Perhaps you have overcome similar challenges before; maybe you have a supportive colleague or friend who will encourage you; you might have extra time to invest in this objective.
- The third step, Options, is where you should think through or write out different ways to make the progress you would like to see. At this stage, it is helpful to come up with at least four different options. Doing this increases your awareness of the possibility of making progress and gives you some backup strategies if some of them don't work.
- The fourth step, Will, involves picking one of the options you chose earlier. Decide which one you think is most likely to lead to success. You can make this decision based on your understanding of yourself and your circumstances. You should commit to one clear way forward by the end of this step.

- The fifth step requires you to be very specific about what you will do and when you will do it. In other words, since you have already committed to a way forward, you now need to write out an action plan. The more specific this is, the better. It is helpful to list your actions and set deadlines for each.
- The final step involves thinking about ensuring that you can sustain the change. Firstly, how will you celebrate your achievement? And then, how can you make sure the new behaviour becomes a habit?

This coaching framework will support you to be more intentional about making progress. With a clear plan of action and a way of monitoring progress, you are more likely to achieve your wellbeing goals.

Option 2: Free Wheel of Health and Wellbeing

Having read this book, reflect on and list what is important to you concerning your health and wellbeing. This may include the following: your relationships, keeping the symptoms of your condition (e.g. multiple sclerosis) at bay, reading books for pleasure, finding some "me" time in the chaos of your family life, getting away on holidays, etc. Now select eight essential things that significantly impact your health and wellbeing, the things without which your wellbeing is compromised. Put each of the eight things into the Free Wheel of Health and Wellbeing (Figure 10.3).

Review each part and reflect on the following:

- How satisfied are you with the first thing, on a scale from 1 to 10 (10 meaning you are delighted)? E.g. the first thing you may have written down are your children. Recently, one of your boys got in trouble for pushing another one at recess. But the other two children are doing well. This is why your satisfaction with this aspect of your life is 7 out of 10.
  - Repeat this process for all other parts.
- Address which part of your wheel would add value to your health and wellbeing. Please do not automatically select the lowest part in the hope that addressing it would resolve an issue. For example, say that your dissatisfaction with the relationship with your spouse is low. However, today is Thursday, and before you come up with a plan on how to improve your satisfaction with your relationship, you would like to be in a better place, so you choose to start with organising some "me" time over the weekend to put you in a good mood. That

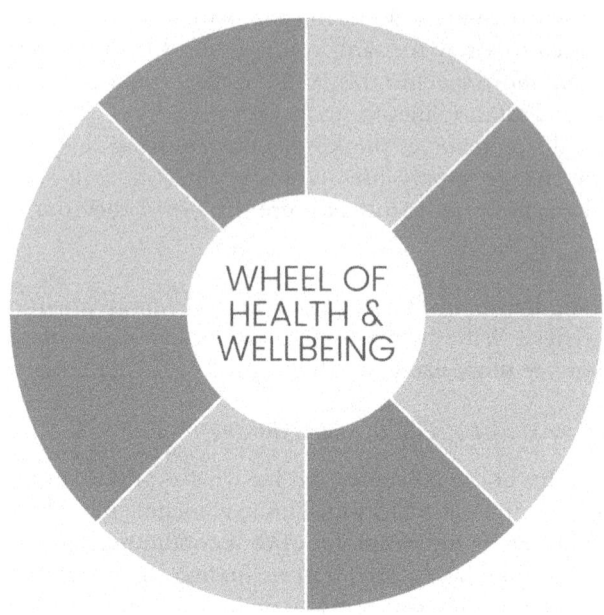

Figure 10.3 Wheel of Health and Wellbeing.

way, next week you will be better able to do something to address the most challenging issue you are facing.
- Now that you have selected one or two parts you would like to address over the next week or so, review the groups of tools in this book and decide which ones could help you become more satisfied with your life. Which ones would you find most helpful at this point?
- Briefly review the tools in this section and decide on one or two tools you want to implement over the next week or a few weeks.
- Please go back to the GROWTH model section, which will guide you through the goal-setting process.

Reflection time

Write down the tools you have selected and the process of goal setting that will help you achieve them. Please use another piece of paper if required.

Find a coach

Executive and life coaching have grown in popularity over the last four decades. Since the start of this century, there has been a growing body of evidence that coaching does *work* because it supports people to set and achieve self-selected goals (Theeboom et al., 2014; de Haan, 2021). It has been shown to support goal attainment, resilience, and wellbeing (Grant, 2003; Grant et al., 2009), even during challenging times like the COVID-19 pandemic (van Nieuwerburgh et al., 2021). Coaching is essentially a process for bringing about behaviour change (Whitmore, 2009); it can be beneficial when adopting new practices. Suppose you are interested in working with someone about health goals. In that case, we recommend finding someone with the relevant experience – a health coach, a wellbeing coach, or a positive psychology coach – who is adequately trained. You can ascertain this by ensuring that they have an appropriate accreditation or university degree.

Find a therapist

Occasionally, you might uncover a more profound issue as you become more aware of your body, behaviour, emotional life, and thinking process. Elements from the past can rear their heads and trigger strong emotional responses. Alternatively, you may already have ongoing mild or moderate depression or anxiety issues. This might be one of the reasons you have sought out this book. You could be going through grief of some kind. Remember that loss is not always about the death of a loved one. We can grieve when we lose a job, end relationships, our adult children leave home, or when we retire. Finally, you might have received a devastating diagnosis that threatens your health or even your life. These diagnoses often come with anger, grief, sadness, a lack of acceptance, and fear. If you have ruled out a physical cause of your anxiety or depression or are dealing with one or many of the issues described, then counselling or psychotherapy might be for you. Awareness is key. Once you become aware of the processes inside you and pay attention to your brain, mind, body, and subconscious, you can begin a plan to emerge with coping skills with the help of a therapist.

First things first: what is the difference between a counsellor and a psychotherapist? These terms can be confusing. Traditionally, counsellors have been those with a diploma in the field who deal with short-term issues such as grief. Psychotherapists usually had a degree and dealt with more complex issues such as long-term mild to moderate depression.

Nowadays, as the field becomes more regulated worldwide, most therapists will have a degree in counselling and psychotherapy and be accredited with a national or international governing body. Make sure you check your national websites, which usually list accredited psychotherapists. This is important.

Second, which therapy is for you? In our experience, this all depends on you, your stage in life, your life experience, and your personality. You might also have to engage in some trial and error. Most therapists will be trained in the art of listening, so that should form the basis of any therapy. Likewise, most modern therapeutic approaches are non-directive and collaborative. You must do most of the work; your therapist will act as a guide. In terms of specific modalities or types of therapy, you will encounter cognitive- and humanistic-based approaches. Cognitive behavioural therapy (CBT) is a practical approach based on the Stoic philosophers of antiquity. We do not have the scope in this book to go into detail. However, the essential elements of CBT involve recognising that you have a core set of beliefs that usually emerge in your childhood. These beliefs can modify your behaviour as an adult. Incidents in life can initiate automatic negative thinking, triggering emotions and behaviour, often linked to your core beliefs. For example, if you had a critical parent, you might emerge from childhood with low self-esteem. If you make a mistake at work as an adult, this could trigger a negative thought: "I am terrible at everything, and I will get fired". This might stop you from working the next day (behaviour change). The result then could be a confirmation of your negative belief, and you get fired. This is an over-simplistic story. In CBT, your therapist will ask you to get a pen and paper and challenge your negative thoughts. Where is the proof that you are terrible? If there is no proof, you incorporate this *fact* into your reality and continuously challenge this type of thinking. You will also realise that you have a choice; you have the power to decide how you respond to thoughts. The result will end this self-perpetuating cycle so that you no longer believe or engage in this type of thinking. Your emotional life will regulate, and your behaviour will become more stable.

Although CBT can be highly effective, it is not for everyone and does not always work (Hofmann et al., 2012). Humanistic therapies,[2] usually referred to as "talk therapies", involve speaking with your therapist in an accessible manner over time. Your therapist might observe changes in body language and tone as you tell your stories. We all have blind spots, psychologically speaking, and your therapist can help you uncover these areas. It might seem simple, but a skilled therapist will often help you uncover underlying issues. It is remarkable how telling your story can make you aware of blind spots that have altered behaviour (including over-eating), thinking, and emotional responses. Your therapist can incorporate a myriad of coping and managing strategies that are often shared with coaching. Sometimes talking is enough. However, usually, we need to develop a personal tool kit to manage these issues. Unfortunately, we do not have the space to cover all types of therapy, including psychoanalysis, Gestalt therapy, choice theory, reality therapy, somatic movement therapy, and schema therapy, among others. These days, most psychotherapists will offer an integrative approach to psychotherapy (Zarbo et al., 2016). Along with your therapist, you can try out different modalities to see which one fits you best.

Notes

1 This is an abridged version of this model, relevant to this book.
2 www.psychologytoday.com/ie/therapy-types/humanistic-therapy

References

Ajzen, I. (1991). The theory of planned behaviour. *Organizational Behaviour and Human Decision Processes*, 50, 179–211.
Bandura, A. (1971). *Social Learning Theory*. General Learning Press.
Bandura, A. (1997). *Self-efficacy: The exercise of control*. W H Freeman/Times Books/Henry Holt & Co.
Campbell, J., & van Nieuwerburgh, C. (2018). *The leader's guide to coaching in schools*. Corwin.
Deci, E. L., & Ryan, R. M. (1985). *Intrinsic motivation and self-determination in human behavior*. Springer Science & Business Media. https://doi.org/10.1007/978-1-4899-2271-7
de Haan, E. (2021). *What works in executive coaching: Understanding outcomes through quantitative research and practice-based evidence*. Routledge.
Frisch, M. B. (2006). *Quality of life therapy: Applying a life satisfaction approach to positive psychology and cognitive therapy*. John Wiley & Sons Ltd.
Grant, A. M. (2003). The impact of life coaching on goal attainment, metacognition and mental health. *Social Behavior and Personality*, 31(3), 253–264.
Grant, A. M., Curtayne, L., & Burton, G. (2009). Executive coaching enhances goal attainment, resilience and workplace wellbeing: A randomised controlled study. *The Journal of Positive Psychology*, 4(5), 396–407.
Hofmann, S. G., Asnaani, A., Vonk, I. J. J., Sawyer, A. T., & Fang, A. (2012). The efficacy of cognitive behavioral therapy: A review of meta-analyses. *Cognitive Therapy and Research*, 36(5), 427–440. doi:10.1007/s10608-012-9476-1
Schwarzer, R. (1992). Self-efficacy in the adoption and maintenance of health behaviors: Theoretical approaches and a new model. In R. Schwarzer (Ed.), *Self-efficacy: Thought control of action* (pp. 217–243). Hemisphere.
Skinner, B. F. (1953). *Science and human behavior*. Macmillan.

Theeboom, T., Beersma, B., & van Vianen, A. E. M. (2014). Does coaching work? A meta-analysis on the effects of coaching on individual level outcomes in an organizational context. *The Journal of Positive Psychology*, *9*, 1–18.

van Nieuwerburgh, C. (2020). *An introduction to coaching skills: A practical guide* (3rd ed.). Sage.

van Nieuwerburgh, C., Barr, M., Fouracres, A. J. S., Moin, T., Brown, C., Holden, C., Lucey, C., & Thomas, P. (2021). Experience of positive psychology coaching while working from home during the covid-19 pandemic: An interpretative phenomenological analysis. *Coaching: An International Journal of Theory, Research and Practice*. Advance online publication. https://doi.org/10.1080/17521882.2021.1897637

Whitmore, J. (1992). *Coaching for performance: A practical guide to growing you own skills*. Nicholas Brealey.

Whitmore, J. (2009). *Coaching for performance: GROWing human potential and purpose: The principles and practice of coaching and leadership* (4th ed.). Nicholas Brealey.

Zarbo, C., Tasca, G. A., Cattafi, F., & Compare, A. (2016). Integrative psychotherapy works. *Frontiers in psychology*, *6*, 2021–2021. doi:10.3389/fpsyg.2015.02021

Conclusion

We wrote this book with you, the reader, in mind. Our aim is to support you in having a healthier future. We don't know who you are. We don't know your life story, what you are proud of, and what you regret. We don't know the joys and struggles you've experienced as you are reading this book today. Nonetheless, as James Joyce wrote in *Ulysses*, we "can't bring back time. Like holding water in your hand". What matters is tomorrow and what you do today and tomorrow to maintain and improve your health. Yesterday has come and gone, and all that is left for us to do is to learn from it, keep looking forward, and keep trying to do better today than we did yesterday. So, enjoy the rest of your life with this book as your health and wellbeing companion. May you be well; may you be healthy; may you be safe!

Index

30x30 Nature Challenge 38

ABCD analysis 86
absorption 162
ABT *see* attention-based training (ABT)
active listening 103
acupressure 26
Adam, H. 185
adrenaline 94
adversity 85–86, 190
aerobics 53–54
affiliative humour 73, 75
ageing 7
agency thinking 179
aggressive humour 73
alcohol 64
altruism 157
amotivation 199
ANS *see* autonomic nervous system (ANS)
anticipation 168; caveat 171; practice variations 169–170; research-based tools 169; wellbeing benefits 170–171
aromatherapy 28
art making, and art therapy 43
art viewing: caveat 128; health benefits 127–128; practice variations 126–127; research-based tools 126; virtual galleries 126
attention-based training (ABT) 33
attitudinal value 132
Aurelius, Marcus 32, 97
autonomic nervous system (ANS) 23
awareness-based meditations 32

beach activities 60
Beghetto, R. A. 42
behavioural change 198–199
behavioural expression 162
"being" mode 23–24
beliefs 86
benefit finding 138; caveats 141; health benefits 140–141; practice variations 140; research-based tools 139–140
benefit reminding 140
best possible health 176–177
best possible self: caveat 178; in future 176; health benefits 177–178; in past 176; practice variations 177; in present 136; research-based tools 176–177
bibliotherapy 89; caveat 91; health benefits 91; practice variations 90; research-based tools 90; and sleep 28
big-C Creativity 42
binge eating 102–103
Blink (Gladwell) 42
Blue Spaces 39, 60–62; caveats 62; diet 64; getting active 60–61; health benefits 61–62; practice variations 61; research-based tools 60–61
Blue Zone Initiative 56, 67
body play 68
Body Scan 32–33
Boehm, J. 160
Bolwerk, A. 45
book club 90
Book of Life 81
book reading 26
breathing 25, 34

214 *Index*

Broaden and Build theory 44, 108
Brockington, G. 184
Bryant, F. B. 161
Burke, J. 26, 54, 95, 97, 178

caffeine, avoiding 26
calming tools: creativity 42–46; green care (gardening/horticulture) 47–49; meditation 32–35; nature 37–40; sleep 24–29
Campion, M. 124
canoeing 60
capitalisation: caveat 152; health benefits 152; practice variations 151–152; research-based tools 151
care of plants *see* gardening (green care)
Carr, A. 86
CBT *see* Cognitive Behavioural Therapy (CBT)
character strengths 113, 115–116
Che Guevara 146–147
children: parents savouring moments 164; sleeping routines 25
Chilton, G. 44
circadian rhythm 26, 27
Clifton Strengths Finder 113
coaching 4, 204–205, 209; GROWTH framework 206–208; practising gratitude 120; quality-of-life (QoL) 145, 204
co-creation 45
Cognitive Behavioural Therapy (CBT) 86, 89, 210
cold-water immersion 61–62
comedy show 74
commensalism 65
community-based exercises 54
compassion 34, 100; caveat 105; characteristics of 101; health benefits 104–105; practice variations 103–104; research-based tools 101–103
Compassionate Mind Foundation 104
competitive altruism 157
concentration-based meditations 32–34
Conner, T. S. 124
conscious exercises 55
consequences 86
consumption, limited 64
coping tools 79; bibliotherapy 89–91; compassion 100–105; expressive writing 80–83; optimism 84–88; stress mindset 93–98

Corda, Alberto 146
cortisol 184
Cotter, Katherine N. 127
count blessings 162
counterfactual thinking 140
COVID pandemic 3
creative value 131
creativity 42–46; caveat 46; health benefits 44–45; and mental illness 45; practice variations 44; research-based tools 43–44
crocheting 44
Croom, A. M. 124
Crum, Alia 96
curiosity 116

daily activity records 53
daily hassles 79
Dalai Lama 157
Daubenmier, J. 65
David Suzuki's Foundation 38
Da Vinci, Leonardo 126
decluttering method 55
defensive pessimism 88
depression, overcoming *see specific tools*
devices, unplugging 26
digital art 126
digital devices 28
disputation 86
distancing 86
distraction 86
"doing" mode 23–24
dragon boat racing 60
dressing up 186
Dunne, Pádraic J. 33
dyslexia 80

eating 64–65, 102
Eisenstaedt, Alfred 146
Ekman, P. 108
electronic devices 26, 28
emerging tools 184–190; harmonious passion 188–189; self-care 185–186; self-reassurance 189–190; social media 187–189; storytelling 184–185
emotions 23; conceptualisations of 108; negative 44, 108, 165, 177; positive emotions 23, 44, 101, 108–109, 111, 127, 148, 167
empathy 70, 91, 100, 104, 190

emulsifiers 64
enclothed cognition 185
energising tools 51–78; blue spaces 60–62; humour 73–76; nutrition 63–67; physical activity 52–57; play 68–71
enjoyment 132
epigenetics 7
exercises 26, 51; breathing relaxation 25; community-based 54; conscious 55; dependence 57; high-intensity 56
experiential value 131
expressive writing 27; caveats 83; health benefits 82–83; practice variations 81–82; research-based tools 80–81
external motivation 199

fairy tale writing 81
"faulty" prospections 167
"feed your brain and gut" 64
feeling-good tools 108; art viewing 126–128; gratitude 118–120; music 122–125; reminiscence 110–112; strengths 113–117
fermented food 64, 76
fictional books 90
fight-or-flight response 93
film savouring 169
flexible optimism 87
fly-fishing 60
folk tales 60
forgiveness 153; caveats 155; health benefits 154–155; practice variations 154; research-based tools 154
Frankl, Victor 97, 131
Fredrickson, Barbara 108, 163
Freud, Sigmund 168
fruits 65
funny things 74
fun shoes 186
future events *see* anticipation

Galinsky, A. D. 185
Gander, F. 11
gardening (green care) 47–49; caveat 49; health benefits 48–49; practice variations 48; research-based tools 48
genes 7–8
gift of time 158
Gilbert, P. 104, 190
Gladwell, Malcolm 42

goal setting: caveat 174–175; health benefits 174; practice variations 173–174; research-based practice 173
good things 118
graffiti 126, 147
gratitude 34; caveats 120; health benefits 120; letter and/or visit 119; list with twist 118–119; practice variations 119–120; research-based tools 118–119; and sleep 28; at work 118
group belonging 135
GROWTH framework 206–207
gut bacteria (microbiome) 66–67

hair styling 186
Hall, A. K. 71
happiness 202
harmonious passion 188–189
health, and wellbeing 5–7; catch and keep 12–13; continuing current practices 13–14; defined 5; enjoyable tools 13; getting dosage right 15; getting social 14–15; and happiness 101; keep going 15–16; meaning-making tools 13; open-minded attitude 14; positive attitude 16; positive psychology and lifestyle medicine 8–10; research-based tools 13; varying activities 14
Health Action Process Approach 198
healthful eating 10
health plan 203–204
Hedonic adaptation 12
Hemingway, Ernest 60
high-intensity exercises 56
Holder, Mark D. 66
hope: caveats 182; health benefits 181; and optimism 179; practice variations 180–181; profiling 180; research-based tools 180
horticulture 47, 48–49
household chores 52–53
humanistic therapies 210
humour 73–76; and burnout 75; caveats 76; health benefits 75–76; research-based tools 74–75

identified motivation 199
improvisation 43
insomnia 25, 29
instant messaging 82

integrated motivation 199
Intense Positive Experience tool 110, 111
intrinsic motivation 199
introjected motivation 199
Isen, Alice 108

job, as calling 114–115
junk foods 64, 103

Kaufman, J. C. 42
kayaking 60
Keech, J. J. 97
Keller, Helen 43
killjoy thinking 162
kin altruism 157
kindness 15, 116, 156–160; caveats 159–160; health benefits 159; perform/observe 158; practice variations 158–159; research-based practice 157–158
King, L. A. 178
Kondo, Marie 55

languishing 3
Latham, G. P. 174
laughter yoga 74
legacy (scarcity): caveats 145; health benefits 144–145; practice variations 144; research-based tools 143–144
letter, from future 173
letter, of forgiveness 154
Levita, L. 124
libido 94
library therapy *see* bibliotherapy
life crafting 132, 133
life longings 170
life meaning 130–131
lifestyle factors 3, 7
lifestyle medicine 8, 9–10
life summary review 143–144
literary fiction 60
literature *see* bibliotherapy
little-c creativity 43
Locke, E. A. 174
logotherapy 131–132, 133
long-term insomnia 25
looking forward to tomorrow 169
loving-kindness meditation 32, 34, 101, 190
Lyubomirsky, S. 160, 178

Maarsingh, B. M. 97
makeup 186
Man's Search for Meaning (Frankl) 97
mantras 32, 33, 123
McCarthy, Catherine 51
meaning exploration 131–134; caveats 133–134; health benefits 133; practice variations 133; research-based tools 131–132
meaningful moments 147
meaning-making tools 130; benefit finding 138–141; exploring meaning 131–134; legacy (scarcity) 143–145; photography 146–148; positive identity 135–137
meditation 104; caveat 35; cultivating compassion and gratitude 34; health benefits 34–35; practice variations 34; research-based tools 32–34; and sleep 28; Zazen (Japanese) 33
Meditations (Aurelius) 97
memory building 161
mental health 5, 25, 49, 56, 98, 155
microbiomes 66–67
mindful eating 65
mindfulness 27, 32–33, 66
mindsets, stress 93–98
mini-c creativity 43
Mona Lisa painting 126
Mongrain, M. 124–125
mood repair 43
Most Feared Obituary 143, 144
motivation 199
Murdoch, Iris 60
musculoskeletal injury 57
music 81; caveats 124–125; health benefits 124; listening to 26; making 123; practice variations 123–124; research-based tools 122–123; before sleep 122–123
mutualism 157
myocardial infarction (heart attack) 57

nature: caveat 40; good things about 37–38; health benefits 39–40; imagining ourselves 38; listening to sound of 38; noticing 38; practice variations 38–39; research-based tools 37–38; visiting 37
nature connectedness 37

nature contact 37
NCDs *see* noncommunicable diseases (NCDs)
Neff, Kristin 104
negative beliefs 167
negative emotions 108
neurotransmitters 66, 105
Niemiec, R. M. 115–116
night worker 26–27
noncommunicable diseases (NCDs) 3
not-so-random acts of kindness 158
nurture 42
nutrition 63–67; caveats 67; health benefits 66–67; practice variations 65; research-based tools 64–65

object play 68
Old Man and the Sea, The (Hemingway) 60
OLIW-model, of playfulness 70
"one door closes, another door opens" 140
open-mindedness 14, 42
Operant Learning Theory 198
optimism 84–88, 179; caveats 87–88; health benefits 87; practice variations 86–87; research-based tools 86
oxytocin 185

parasympathetic systems 23–24
passion 188–189
past events, remembering 162
pathway thinking 179
Pawelski, James O. 127
Penn Resiliency programme 11, 86
PERMA Profiler 70
personality trait 85
pessimism 85, 199
photography 39, 146–148; caveats 148; health benefits 148; practice variations 147–148; research-based tools 147
physical activity 10, 56; caveats 57; health benefits 56–57; practice variations 54–55; research-based tools 52–54
Picture This! research 147
playfulness 44, 68–71; in adults 68, 71; caveats 71; health benefits 70–71; OLIW-model of 70; practice variations 70; research-based tools 69; stimulating 69
playlist 69
poor evaluation 167
poor potential 167
positive attitude 16
positive change 202
positive emotions 23, 44, 108–109
positive experiences 110, 161
positive identity: caveats 137; health benefits 137; practice variations 136–137; research-based tools 135–136
positive introduction 136
positive legacy 143, 144
positive mental time travel 169
positive psychology 8–12, 66, 113
Positive Psychology at the Movies (Niemiec & Wedding) 116
positive psychology interventions (PPIs) 11
positive psychotherapy 144
positive realism 87
positivity resonance 163
post-traumatic growth (PTG) 138–139, 141
post-traumatic stress disorder 79, 82
PPIs *see* positive psychology interventions (PPIs)
prayer chanting 123
Present Perfect (Somov) 90
pre-shift nap 26
pro-c creativity 43
pro-social spending 158
prospecting tools 167; anticipation 168–171; best possible self 176–178; goal setting 173–175; hope 179–182
prospective writing 169
psychological blind spots 210
PTG *see* post-traumatic growth (PTG)
punishment 198
PURE (purpose/understanding/responsibility/enjoyment) principles 132
purpose 132

quality-of-life therapy 144, 204

radio discussions 123
random acts, of kindness 157

Random Acts of Kindness Foundation 158
RCT (randomised controlled trial) 65
realism 201
reciprocal altruism 157
reflective body language 103
reflective writing 177
relationship tools 150; capitalisation 151–152; forgiveness 153–155; forming/maintaining 10; kindness 156–160; savouring relationships 161–165
reminiscence: caveat 112; health benefits 111–112; practice variations 111; research-based tools 110
responsibility 132
risky substances, avoiding 11
Round, J. 178

sailing 60
saliva production 24, 184
Salvador Mundi painting 126
savouring relationships 161; caveat 164–165; child 163; health benefits 163–164; practice variations 163; research-based tools 162–163; for young people 162–163
scarcity: caveats 145; health benefits 144–145; practice variations 144; research-based tools 143–144
Schwarz, Tony 51
scuba diving 60
seagazing 61
Seanchaí (storytellers) 184
Sea, the Sea, The (Murdoch) 60
self-affirmation 135–136
self-care 185–186
self-compassion 102, 103, 190
self-concordance model 174
self-congratulations 162
self-criticism 190
self-defeating humour 74
self-deprecating jokes 75
self-determination theory 199
self-efficacy 198
self-enhancing humour 73, 75
self-help industry 89–90
self-reassurance 189–190
Seligman, Martin 85, 86, 114, 118, 136, 143
sensory perceptual sharpening 162

Sergeant, S. 124–125
serotonin 66
seven humour habits programme 75
shame 104–105
shared connection 163
Sheldon, K. M. 160, 178
Sherman, A. 126–127
short-term insomnia 25
sickness behaviour 94
signature strengths 114
skygazing 61
sleep 24–29; caveat 29; disturbances 29; health benefits 28–29; improving 11; music before 122–123; practice variations 27; research-based tools 25–27
Sloan, D. M. 82
SMART goals 204
Social Cognitive Theory 198
social identity 135–136, 137
Social Learning Theory 198
social media 81, 187–189
social play 14–15, 68
Socratic questioning 86–87
Somov, Pavel 90
Stanford Mind and Body Lab 96
Steger, M. F. 147
storytelling 44, 184–185
strengths: assessment 114; caveat 116–117; family contract 115; health benefits 116; lesser 114; practice variations 115–116; research-based tools 114–115
Strengths Profile 113
stress: management 10; overcoming with humour 74
stress mindset 93–98; caveat 98; enhancing/debilitating 95, 97–98; health benefits 97–98; practice variations 96–97; research-based tools 96
Stress Mindset Measure questionnaire 97
suicides 3
support group 188
surfing 60
swimming 60
sympathetic systems 23–24

temporal awareness 162
temporal scarcity 144

Theory of Planned Behaviour 198
therapist 209–211
transtheoretical model 199
traumas 79

understanding 132
uplifting music 122, 124

Vaillant, G. E. 133
van Beethoven, Ludwig 122
Van Bulck, L. 135
vblog 81
vegetables 65
Veroff, J. 161
VIA Character Strengths Questionnaire 113, 115
volunteering 102
Von Humboldt, Wilhelm 51

walk-and-talk therapy 38
walking 39–40
watching comedy 74
water sports 60–61
Wedding, D. 115–116

Weldon, C. 71
wellbeing 4; and health 5–7; psychological and physiological effects 11–12
"what might have been" 140, 141
Wheel of Health and Wellbeing 205–208
WHO *see* World Health Organisation (WHO)
Wilkinson, R. 44
Wing, J. F. 111
winter swimming 61
wishful thinking 179
Wong, P. 131
World Health Organisation (WHO): art viewing and art making 126; defines health 5; physical activity 52; sleep 24
writing therapy (WT) 80
WT *see* writing therapy (WT)
WWW (want went well) activity 120

yoga 53–54, 123
yoghurt 64

Zazen (Japanese) sitting meditation 33

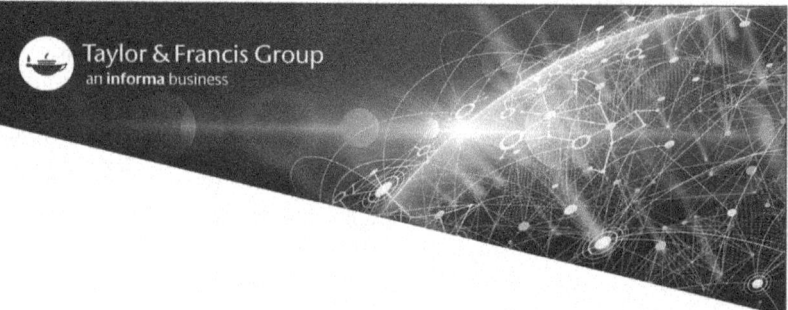